Organ Failure in Critical Illness

Guest Editor

TIMOTHY B. HACKETT, DVM, MS

VETERINARY CLINICS OF NORTH AMERICA: SMALL ANIMAL PRACTICE

www.vetsmall.theclinics.com

July 2011 • Volume 41 • Number 4

SAUNDERS an imprint of ELSEVIER, Inc.

W.B. SAUNDERS COMPANY
A Division of Elsevier Inc.

1600 John F. Kennedy Blvd. ● Suite 1800 ● Philadelphia, PA 19103-2899
http://www.vetsmall.theclinics.com

VETERINARY CLINICS OF NORTH AMERICA: SMALL ANIMAL PRACTICE Volume 41, Number 4
July 2011 ISSN 0195-5616, ISBN-13: 978-1-4557-1162-8

Editor: John Vassallo; j.vassallo@elsevier.com

Veterinary Clinics of North America: Small Animal Practice (ISSN 0195-5616) is published bimonthly (For Post Office use only: volume 41 issue 4 of 6) by Elsevier Inc., 360 Park Avenue South, New York, NY 10010-1710. Months of issue are January, March, May, July, September, and November. Business and Editorial Offices: 1600 John F. Kennedy Blvd., Ste. 1800, Philadelphia, PA 19103-2899. Customer Service Office: 3251 Riverport Lane, Maryland Heights, MO 63043. Periodicals postage paid at New York, NY and additional mailing offices. Subscription prices are $262.00 per year (domestic individuals), $427.00 per year (domestic institutions), $128.00 per year (domestic students/residents), $347.00 per year (Canadian individuals), $525.00 per year (Canadian institutions), $385.00 per year (international individuals), $525.00 per year (international institutions), and $186.00 per year (international and Canadian students/residents). To receive student/resident rate, orders must be accompanied by name of affiliated institution, date of term, and the *signature* of program/residency coordinator on institution letterhead. Orders will be billed at individual rate until proof of status is received. Foreign air speed delivery is included in all *Clinics* subscription prices. All prices are subject to change without notice. **POSTMASTER:** Send address changes to *Veterinary Clinics of North America: Small Animal Practice*, Elsevier Health Sciences Division, Subscription Customer Service, 3251 Riverport Lane, Maryland Heights, MO 63043. Customer Service (orders, claims, online, change of address): Elsevier Periodicals Customer Service, Elsevier Health Sciences Division Subscription Customer Service 3251 Riverport Lane Maryland Heights, MO 63043. Tel: 1-800-654-2452 (U.S. and Canada); 314-447-8871 (outside U.S. and Canada). Fax: 314-447-8029. E-mail: journalscustomerservice-usa@elsevier.com (for print support); journalsonlinesupport-usa@elsevier.com (for online support).

Reprints. For copies of 100 or more of articles in this publication, please contact the Commercial Reprints Department, Elsevier Inc., 360 Park Avenue South, New York, NY 10010-1710. Tel.: 212-633-3812; Fax: 212-462-1935; E-mail: reprints@elsevier.com.

Veterinary Clinics of North America: Small Animal Practice is also published in Japanese by Inter Zoo Publishing Co., Ltd., Aoyama Crystal-Bldg 5F, 3-5-12 Kitaaoyama, Minato-ku, Tokyo 107-0061, Japan.

Veterinary Clinics of North America: Small Animal Practice is covered in *Current Contents/Agriculture, Biology and Environmental Sciences, Science Citation Index, ASCA, MEDLINE/PubMed (Index Medicus), Excerpta Medica,* and *BIOSIS.*

Printed in the United States of America.

Contributors

GUEST EDITOR

TIMOTHY B. HACKETT, DVM, MS
Diplomate, American College of Veterinary Emergency and Critical Care;
Professor of Emergency and Critical Care Medicine, Department of Clinical Sciences,
Colorado State University, Fort Collins, Colorado

AUTHORS

BENJAMIN M. BRAINARD, VMD
Diplomate, American College of Veterinary Anesthesiologists; Diplomate,
American College of Veterinary Emergency and Critical Care; Associate Professor,
Critical Care, Department of Small Animal Medicine and Surgery, University of
Georgia, Athens, Georgia

ANDREW J. BROWN, MA VetMB, MRCVS
Diplomate, American College of Veterinary Emergency and Critical Care,
VetsNow Referral Hospital, Glasgow, Scotland, United Kingdom

BARRET J. BULMER, DVM, MS
Diplomate, American College of Veterinary Internal Medicine-Cardiology;
Clinical Assistant Professor, Department of Clinical Sciences, Cummings
School of Veterinary Medicine at Tufts University, North Grafton, Massachusetts

AMY L. BUTLER, DVM, MS
Diplomate, American College of Veterinary Emergency and Critical Care;
Director of Emergency and Critical Care, Veterinary Referral and Emergency Center,
Clarks Summit, Pennsylvania

VICKI LYNNE CAMPBELL, DVM
Diplomate, American College of Veterinary Anesthesiologists; Diplomate,
American College of Veterinary Emergency and Critical Care; Associate Professor of
Veterinary Emergency and Critical Care, Department of Clinical Sciences,
Colorado State University, Fort Collins, Colorado

DANIEL L. GUSTAFSON, PhD
Associate Professor of Clinical Pharmacology and Animal Cancer Center;
Director of Research, Department of Clinical Sciences, Colorado State University,
Fort Collins, Colorado

EILEEN S. HACKETT, DVM, MS
Diplomate, American College of Veterinary Emergency and Critical Care; Diplomate,
American College of Veterinary Surgeons; Assistant Professor of Surgery and Critical
Care, Department of Clinical Sciences, Colorado State University, Fort Collins, Colorado

TIMOTHY B. HACKETT, DVM, MS
Diplomate, American College of Veterinary Emergency and Critical Care;
Professor of Emergency and Critical Care Medicine, Department of Clinical Sciences,
Colorado State University, Fort Collins, Colorado

KATHARINE F. LUNN, BVMS, MS, PhD, MRCVS
Diplomate, American College of Veterinary Internal Medicine; Assistant Professor,
Small Animal Internal Medicine, Department of Clinical Sciences, Colorado State
University, Fort Collins, Colorado

LINDA G. MARTIN, DVM, MS
Diplomate, American College of Veterinary Emergency and Critical Care;
Associate Professor of Emergency and Critical Care Medicine, College of Veterinary
Medicine, Auburn University; Acting Director, Small Animal Intensive Care Unit,
Auburn University Small Animal Teaching Hospital, Auburn, Alabama

KELLY W. MCCORD, DVM, MS
Senior Resident, Small Animal Internal Medicine, Department of Clinical Sciences,
James L. Voss Veterinary Teaching Hospital, Colorado State University,
Fort Collins, Colorado

CRAIG B. WEBB, PhD, DVM
Diplomate, American College of Veterinary Internal Medicine;
Associate Professor and Head of Small Animal Internal Medicine,
Department of Clinical Sciences, James L. Voss Veterinary Teaching Hospital,
Colorado State University, Fort Collins, Colorado

Contents

Preface: Organ Failure in Critical Illness   ix

Timothy B. Hackett

Introduction to Multiple Organ Dysfunction and Failure   **703**

Timothy B. Hackett

Multiple organ failure and multiple organ dysfunction syndrome (MODS) were first recognized as undesirable complications of advancements in emergency and critical care. MODS remains the leading cause of death and resource expenditure in human intensive care units. MODS has been documented in small animal veterinary patients raising similar concerns. The understanding of the pathogenesis of MODS has evolved from uncontrolled infection to uncontrolled inflammation. Management is primarily through supportive care, early and aggressive monitoring of organ function, and intensive care nursing. Tissue hypoxia, microvascular thrombosis, increased vascular permeability, and disrupted cell-cell communication are prominent features of MODS.

Respiratory Complications in Critical Illness of Small Animals   **709**

Vicki Lynne Campbell

The percentage of emergency patients with respiratory problems treated at veterinary emergency and critical care facilities is poorly defined. Regardless of whether an animal has a primary lung disease or develops a secondary lung disease during hospitalization, acute respiratory distress syndrome (ARDS) is a common sequela to the failing lung. ARDS is a frequent sequela to sepsis, systemic inflammatory response (SIRS), and disseminated intravascular coagulation and is frequently the pulmonary manifestation of multiple organ dysfunction syndrome (MODS). ARDS, acute lung injury, SIRS, sepsis, and MODS are serious syndromes with grave consequences. Understanding the pathophysiology and consequences of these syndromes is imperative to early recognition.

Cardiovascular Dysfunction in Sepsis and Critical Illness   **717**

Barret J. Bulmer

Myocardial dysfunction is commonly encountered in humans, and presumably in dogs with sepsis and critical illness. This dysfunction contributes to increased mortality. With management of the underlying diseases and an understanding of the processes contributing to myocardial dysfunction, steps may be taken to mitigate the consequences of cardiac impairment. Clinical findings, proposed pathophysiologic mechanisms, and current treatment considerations are discussed. Further study is needed to find practical ways to identify myocardial dysfunction and to determine whether timed interventions intended to augment cardiac performance will reduce mortality in this patient population.

The Kidney in Critically Ill Small Animals   **727**

Katharine F. Lunn

> Critically ill animals may have preexisting renal disease or develop acute
> kidney injury as a consequence of their presenting complaint. Age, concur-
> rent medical therapy, electrolyte and fluid imbalances, and exposure to
> potential nephrotoxicants are factors that predispose to acute kidney
> injury. Many risk factors are correctable or manageable, and these should
> be addressed whenever possible. Measurement of serum creatinine is
> insensitive for the detection of acute kidney injury, and clinicians should
> consider assessment of other parameters such as urine output, urinalysis,
> and urine chemistry results. A stepwise approach for management of
> acute kidney injury in small animal patients is outlined.

Hepatic Dysfunction   **745**

Kelly W. McCord and Craig B. Webb

> This article reviews the common pathophysiology that constitutes hepatic
> dysfunction, regardless of the inciting cause. The systemic consequences
> of liver failure and the impact of this condition on other organ systems are
> highlighted. The diagnostic tests available for determining the cause and
> extent of liver dysfunction are outlined, treatment strategies aimed at sup-
> porting hepatic health and recovery are discussed, and prognosis is briefly
> covered. The article emphasizes the fact that because of the central role of
> the liver in maintaining normal systemic homeostasis, hepatic dysfunction
> cannot be effectively addressed as an isolated entity.

Gastrointestinal Complications of Critical Illness in Small Animals   **759**

Timothy B. Hackett

> The gastrointestinal (GI) tract is one of the shock organs in dogs. GI dys-
> function in critically ill veterinary patients manifests in mild problems
> such as hypomotility, anorexia, and nausea to more serious problems
> such as intractable vomiting, severe diarrhea, and septicemia. Septicemia
> is a serious complication of GI dysfunction because intestinal flora gains
> access to a patient's bloodstream, leading to infections in other organ
> systems and a systemic inflammatory response. The therapy for GI dys-
> function is mainly supportive, treating nausea and dehydration although
> supporting the ailing GI tract with adequate enteral nutrition and, in
> some cases, dietary supplements and antibiotics.

Critical Illness-Related Corticosteroid Insufficiency in Small Animals   **767**

Linda G. Martin

> Critical illness-related corticosteroid insufficiency (CIRCI) describes endo-
> crine abnormalities associated with illness. CIRCI is characterized by an
> inadequate production of cortisol in relation to an increased demand dur-
> ing periods of severe stress, particularly in critical illnesses such as sepsis
> or septic shock. A hallmark sign of CIRCI is hypotension refractory to fluid
> resuscitation, requiring vasopressor therapy. Corticosteroid treatment can
> be indicated in patients with CIRCI. This article reviews the physiology and
> pathophysiology of the corticosteroid response to critical illness and the
> incidence, clinical features, diagnosis, and treatment of CIRCI.

Defects in Coagulation Encountered in Small Animal Critical Care 783

Benjamin M. Brainard and Andrew J. Brown

Critically ill small animals are at risk for developing coagulation abnormalities. The processes of inflammation and coagulation are intertwined, and severe inflammation can lead to disturbances of coagulation. Severe coagulation dysfunction is associated with increased morbidity and mortality. Pathophysiology, diagnosis, and treatment of coagulation dysfunction are discussed. Defects in coagulation in small animal patients are complex and a consensus on diagnosis and treatment has yet to be reached.

Alterations of Drug Metabolism in Critically Ill Animals 805

Eileen S. Hackett and Daniel L. Gustafson

Critically ill animals are by nature a diverse group with multiple presenting complaints and differing levels of organ function. Pharmacokinetics and pharmacodynamics of administered compounds are affected both by the disease processes and by the interventions of the treating veterinarian. Polypharmacy is not an exception but a rule within this caseload. Basic principles of pharmacology allow for safe and effective administration of pharmaceuticals, especially in the critically ill. Future research evaluating the pharmacokinetics and pharmacodynamics of drugs important in the management of critically ill animals is imperative, and will allow evidence-based dose modification.

Goal-Directed Therapy in Small Animal Critical Illness 817

Amy L. Butler

Monitoring critically ill patients can be a daunting task even for experienced clinicians. Goal-directed therapy is a technique involving intensive monitoring and aggressive management of hemodynamics in patients with high risk of morbidity and mortality. The aim of goal-directed therapy is to ensure adequate tissue oxygenation and survival. This article reviews commonly used diagnostics in critical care medicine and what the information gathered signifies and discusses clinical decision making on the basis of diagnostic test results. One example is early goal-directed therapy for severe sepsis and septic shock. The components and application of goals in early goal-directed therapy are discussed.

Index 839

FORTHCOMING ISSUES

September 2011
Surgical Complications
Christopher A. Adin, DVM,
Guest Editor

November 2011
Suburban Companion Animal Medicine:
Infectious, Toxicological and Parasitic
Diseases
Sanjay Kapil, DVM, PhD,
Guest Editor

January 2012
Small Animal Toxicology
Stephen B. Hooser, DVM, PhD
and Safdar A. Khan, DVM, MS, PhD,
Guest Editors

RECENT ISSUES

May 2011
Palliative Medicine and Hospice Care
Tamara S. Shearer, DVM,
Guest Editor

March 2011
Chronic Intestinal Diseases of Dogs and Cats
Frédéric P. Gaschen, Dr med vet, Dr habil,
Guest Editor

January 2011
Kidney Diseases and Renal Replacement
Therapies
Mark J. Acierno, MBA, DVM and
Mary Anna Labato, DVM, *Guest Editors*

RELATED INTEREST

Veterinary Clinics of North America: Exotic Animal Practice
May 2011 (Vol. 14, No. 2)
The Exotic Animal Respiratory System
Susan E. Orosz, PhD, DVM, Dipl. ABVP—Avian, Dipl. ECZM—Avian and Cathy A.
Johnson-Delaney, DVM, Dipl. ABVP—Avian and Exotic Companion Mammal,
Guest Editors

THE CLINICS ARE NOW AVAILABLE ONLINE!

Access your subscription at:
www.theclinics.com

Preface

Organ Failure in Critical Illness

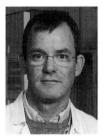

Timothy B. Hackett, DVM, MS
Guest Editor

This issue of *Veterinary Clinics of North America: Small Animal Practice* is devoted to a systems-based review of organ dysfunction seen in our most critical patients. With advances in trauma and emergency care, patients surviving previously fatal problems now succumb to the failure of one or more major systems. While devastating, multiple organ failure is really a disease of success. A single patient may suffer altered function in any or all of the systems discussed in this text. My goal in bringing together these experts and articles is to provide a single reference to review causes, diagnosis, management, and prevention of vital organ dysfunction in small animals. I hope this will be a useful reference for small animal practitioners managing these complex cases.

After an introduction on the history, epidemiology, and understanding of organ failure, experts discuss individual organ systems. The authors are all practicing specialists who see and manage these cases in their respective practices. I will admit to a personal bias toward the respiratory system. Respiratory failure and inadequate tissue oxygenation are leading causes of the failure of other organ systems. Dr Campbell starts off with important insight into the acute respiratory distress syndrome and respiratory failure in the critically ill. While hypotension and inadequate cardiac output as causes of organ failure are discussed in nearly every article, Dr Bulmer's article on cardiac dysfunction highlights the myocardial changes seen in the septic and systemically ill. The kidney and liver are often the most obvious systems failures we associate with critical illness. Dr Lunn presents the causes and management of acute renal failure and Drs McCord and Webb discuss the manifestations and management of hepatic failure. The role of the gastrointestinal tract in critical illness including the signs and consequences of gastrointestinal failure are also discussed.

Moving away from classic organ systems, Dr Martin discusses the important role of the adrenal gland in the body's response to stress. Her article focuses on the recognition and management of adrenal insufficiency associated with critical illness.

Vet Clin Small Anim 41 (2011) ix–x
doi:10.1016/j.cvsm.2011.05.014
0195-5616/11/$ – see front matter © 2011 Elsevier Inc. All rights reserved.

vetsmall.theclinics.com

Drs Brainard and Brown nicely summarize the challenges of managing coagulation defects associated with so many serious conditions. Drs Hackett and Gustafson review altered drug metabolism in critical illness, bringing the clinical pharmacologist's perspective to these heavily medicated patients. Dr Butler rounds out this issue with an overview of goal-directed therapy. Her article gives many practical treatment options for managing high-risk patients.

It has been my privilege to put together this issue. I want to thank the section authors for their time and dedication. I also want to thank Mr John Vassallo and his staff at Saunders/Elsevier for their patience and assistance in compiling this reference. Critical care medicine is constantly evolving. I look forward to the discovery and dissemination of practical solutions to these all too common complications.

Timothy B. Hackett, DVM, MS
Department of Clinical Sciences
Colorado State University
300 West Drake Road
Fort Collins, CO 80523, USA

E-mail address:
Tim.Hackett@colostate.edu

Introduction to Multiple Organ Dysfunction and Failure

Timothy B. Hackett, DVM, MS

KEYWORDS

- MODS • MOF • SIRS • Sepsis • Organ failure

HISTORY AND DEFINITIONS

Multiple organ failure (MOF) was first recognized in human patients with shock in the 1960s. Patients successfully resuscitated often went on to die from a complex disease process that was characterized by the progressive, and usually irreversible, failure of several organs. The condition is an unintended consequence of improved initial success rates in resuscitation. This condition is also true in veterinary medicine. Patients that would have died earlier are surviving the initial insult and succumbing to a series of medical complications. One of the first uses of the term MOF came in 1975, and the term was used to describe the progressive failure of many or all systems after an overwhelming injury or operation. Baue[1] emphasized that death during critical illness was the consequence of the interaction of multiple failing organs and that injury to 1 organ system could cause dysfunction of others.

With advances in critical care medicine, the term MOF is less appropriate because it implies a pessimistic outcome. Failure is too simplistic a term for the clinical and functional derangements observed among major organ systems in the intensively monitored patient. One of the main objectives of intensive critical care medicine is to identify and correct the causes of organ dysfunction before the change becomes irreversible. Therefore, a better term is multiple organ dysfunction syndrome (MODS). MODS defines the progressive, but potentially reversible, dysfunction of 2 or more organ systems after acute life-threatening disruption of systemic homeostasis.[2] The recognition of organ dysfunction in veterinary medicine has paralleled the human experience. In 1989, one of the first collaborative efforts of the Charter Diplomates of the American College of Veterinary Emergency and Critical Care was the *Veterinary Clinics of North America* devoted to critical care. In this journal, investigators discussed MOF,

The author has nothing to disclose.
Department of Clinical Sciences, Colorado State University, 300 West Drake Road, Fort Collins, CO 80523, USA
E-mail address: Tim.Hackett@colostate.edu

Vet Clin Small Anim 41 (2011) 703–707
doi:10.1016/j.cvsm.2011.05.003
0195-5616/11/$ – see front matter © 2011 Elsevier Inc. All rights reserved.

MODS, and the ways that advanced monitoring by highly trained clinicians, which could reduce the morbidity and mortality of systemic disease.[3]

EPIDEMIOLOGY

In 1989, MODS was found to complicate 15% of all intensive care unit (ICU) admissions. MODS was identified as the principal cause of death in patients in the ICU, and the mortality rate increased with the number of acquired problems with major organ systems.[4] More than 40 years after its initial description, MODS remains the leading cause of death in critically ill human patients.[5] In 2000, MODS was reported to be responsible for 50% to 80% of ICU deaths, and patients who develop MODS had a 20 times higher mortality rate and a 2 times longer hospitalization compared with unaffected patients.[6] Although the number of cases of MODS seems to be on the rise, it is important to remember that MODS is a consequence of improved primary care.

It has been recognized that there is a correlation with the number of dysfunctional organ systems and overall mortality. In 1980, the mortality rate associated with failure of a single organ was 30%; the mortality rate associated with the failure of 4 or more organs was 100%.[7] Dysfunction of some organ systems carries a poorer overall prognosis than others. For example, pulmonary failure occurs more often with the dysfunction of at least one other system and the mortality rate of acute respiratory failure is determined by the severity of the nonpulmonary organ dysfunction.[8] A veterinary clinical report in 2010 of 114 dogs with sepsis found that the overall mortality rate was 70% with MODS and 25% for those with only dysfunction of 1 organ system. The odds ratio for the risk of death in this study increased as the number of dysfunctional organ systems increased, and dysfunction of either the respiratory, cardiovascular, renal, or coagulation system was independently associated with a significantly increased odds of death.[9]

PATHOPHYSIOLOGY

MODS was first thought to be caused by infection until it was observed during autopsies that a demonstrated source of infection was not identified; either infection was never present or MODS progressed despite successful surgical and antimicrobial therapy.[10] Around the same time, it was also reported that trauma patients with MODS usually were not infected.[11] Still another report found that infectious complications could develop both before and after MODS.[12] The observation that infection could cause MODS, but was not required, provided the groundwork for the concept of systemic activation and dysregulation of the inflammatory cascade causing the organ dysfunction and failure.[11] The combined effect of inappropriate host defense response and the dysregulation of the immune and systemic inflammatory responses leads to cell injury and tissue and organ damage.[13]

Although noninfectious systemic disorders can activate the cascade of events resulting in organ dysfunction, gram-negative endotoxemia has been one of the most studied.[4] Gram-negative endotoxin is a lipopolysaccharide (LPS) in the outer cell wall. LPS interacts with vascular endothelial cells, neutrophils, platelets, lymphocytes, macrophages, and other cells to release the inflammatory cytokines required to initiate the host's inflammatory response.[14] Tumor necrosis factor α (TNF-α) and isoforms of interleukin (IL) 1 are important early proinflammatory mediators of the host response to injury and have multiple effects that contribute to MODS. Other products of inflammation, including eicosanoid metabolites of the arachidonic acid cascade, platelet activating factor, and nitric oxide, mediate the actions of TNF-α and both IL-1α and IL-1β.[15] Progression from an initial local response to injury to MODS depends on the balance (or lack thereof) between the proinflammatory cytokines and their antiinflammatory counterparts (IL-4, IL-6, IL-10, granulocyte colony-stimulating factor).[16] When these mediators reach systemic levels, what normally functions to contain infection may culminate in progressive cardiopulmonary dysfunction, hypotension, increased vascular permeability, impaired tissue perfusion, organ dysfunction, and death.

Systemic insults leading to MODS have been described by several models.[17] According to the 1-hit model, organ failure develops as the direct result of a massive initial insult such as major trauma or a septic peritonitis. The 2-hit model describes multiple insults, usually isolated over a short period of hours to days. A priming insult such as major trauma is followed by another systemic insult such as aspiration pneumonia. The second hit induces an exaggerated inflammatory response and immune dysfunction and, eventually, MODS. The third model, the sustained-hit model, postulates that a continuous smoldering insult, such as drug-resistant bacterial infection, can both cause and sustain MODS. In reality, any combination of these mechanisms may result in MODS.[17]

In recognition of the importance of systemic inflammation, an American College of Chest Physicians and Society of Critical Care Medicine consensus statement put forth diagnostic criteria for the systemic inflammatory response syndrome (SIRS) in 1992.[18] Eventually, the hypothesis was refined such that a hypodynamic, excessive, or otherwise dysfunctional immune response was said to be the principal cause of organ damage, rather than the direct cytotoxicity of invading microorganisms, whereby any stressor that activates systemic inflammation may precipitate SIRS, thus posing a risk for MODS.[5] The definition of SIRS was modified for companion animals and included 2 of the following:

1. Temperature greater than 103.5°C or less than 100°F
2. Heart rate greater than 160 beats per minute (bpm) in dogs and greater than 250 bpm in cats
3. Respiratory rate greater than 20 breaths per minute or $PaCO_2$ less than 32 mm Hg
4. White blood cell count greater than 12,000 cells/μL, lesser than 4000 cells/μL, or more than 10% bands.[19]

CLINICAL SCORING SYSTEMS

Although azotemia and oliguria indicate renal dysfunction, coma scores objectively define neurologic impairment and bilirubin or bile acid levels can help discern functional hepatic insufficiency; other organ systems have multiple functions that are not subject to objective clinical measurements. Although a universal classification system is lacking, numerous human and veterinary scoring systems have been devised to objectively rank a patient's severity of disease. One of the first classification systems was the Acute Physiology and Chronic Health Evaluation II scoring system.[4] Numerous other systems are in use at present, and some human systems, such as the Multiple Organ Dysfunction Score and the Sequential Organ Failure Assessment, have been applied in small animal clinical research.[9,20] A veterinary scoring system, the Survival Prediction Index, has also been evaluated and validated in clinical small animal patients.[21] Although useful to objectively compare the degree of physiologic derangements and stratify cases for the purpose of research and statistical evaluation, these scoring systems do not address the pathogenic significance of specific organ dysfunctions in an individual patient.

DIAGNOSTIC EVALUATION

Serial monitoring of the major organ systems is the basis of critical care medicine and is necessary to detect early derangements in function. Monitoring to evaluate the function of multiple organ systems should include comprehensive diagnostic tests. A complete blood cell count, arterial blood gas analysis, serum biochemical profile, and tests of coagulation function should be obtained. In addition to the chemistry analysis of blood urea nitrogen and creatinine, urine should be checked for inflammatory cells, casts, and protein. Tissue perfusion can be assessed subjectively by examining mucous membranes. Color and capillary refill times provide information about the adequacy of cardiac output and the state of peripheral vascular resistance. More objective assessment of perfusion includes serum creatinine and blood lactate.

Because sepsis is a leading cause of SIRS, efforts should be made to identify infectious causes. Suspicion of sepsis or septic shock requires that diagnostic material be collected immediately and appropriate monitoring and therapeutic procedures instituted. Distinguishing sepsis from SIRS requires careful exclusion. Every effort should be made to identify and treat potential sources of infection. Areas of concern include the urinary tract, reproductive tract, abdominal cavity, respiratory tract, gingiva, and heart valves. Investigating possible sources of infection requires a thorough medical history concerning gastrointestinal signs, reproductive status (neutered, recent estrus), abnormal urination, recurrent infections, travel, or a recent dentistry. A complete physical examination is performed with attention to oral examination, cardiac and thoracic auscultations, and abdominal palpation. Blood samples are drawn for complete blood cell count; serum biochemical profile; coagulation testing; and rickettsial, fungal, and immune testings if indicated. Urine is collected for analysis and culture. Blood cultures should be taken from the jugular vein after surgically preparing the skin. Because blood cultures can have a low yield, multiple samples should be taken 15 minutes to 1 hour apart ideally during peak increases in body temperature. Antibiotic administration should be withheld until samples are collected, but there should not be any significant delay in starting therapy.

Radiographs and ultrasonographic results of the abdomen may reveal masses, organomegaly or fluid-filled lesions. Loss of abdominal detail suggests abdominal fluid. Radiographs of the chest and echocardiography help evaluate the heart and lungs. With any evidence of fluid in the chest or abdomen, sterile collection for fluid analysis and culture should be performed. If interstitial changes in the lung fields and clinical findings support possible pulmonary disease, bronchoscopy or a transtracheal wash may provide samples for a diagnosis.

SUMMARY

MODS is a disease seen only after successful resuscitation of a serious event. As clinical skills advance and efforts to manage the sickest animal patients are successful, patients with organ dysfunction continue to present a challenge. Meeting this challenge requires excellent teamwork and communication between clinicians and nursing staff so that each individual patient is monitored closely for evidence of altered organ function. To this end, we should continue to improve our monitoring skills and either expand the hours of coverage or refer these critical patients to 24-hour facilities. Current treatment of MODS remains supportive. Once organ system dysfunction is identified, specific steps can be taken to support those systems while the patient recovers from the primary hit. The appropriate and individualized use of fluids, blood transfusions, supplemental oxygen, and drugs to support the delivery of oxygen to the patient's tissues and maintain organ health becomes the primary concern. Clinicians and researchers should continue to work together to further understand MODS and develop new strategies to address this syndrome.

REFERENCES

1. Baue AE. Multiple, progressive, or sequential systems failure: a syndrome of the 1970s. Arch Surg 1975;110:779–81.
2. Ashbaugh DG, Bigelow DB, Petty TL, et al. Acute respiratory distress in adults. Lancet 1967;2:319–23.
3. Kirby R, Stamp GL, editors. Critical care. Vet Clin North Am Small Anim Pract 1989;19(6).
4. Knaus WA, Wagner DP. Multiple systems organ failure: epidemiology and prognosis. Crit Care Clin 1989;5:221–32.
5. Barie PS, Hydo LJ, Pieracci FM, et al. Multiple organ dysfunction syndrome in critical surgical illness. Surg Infect 2009;10:369–77.
6. Barie PS, Hydo LJ. Epidemiology of multiple organ dysfunction syndrome in critical surgical illness. Surg Infect 2000;1:173–83.
7. Fry DE, Fulton RL, Polk HC Jr. Multiple system organ failure: the role of uncontrolled infection. Arch Surg 1980;115:136–40.
8. Schwartz DB, Bone RC, Balk RA, et al. Hepatic dysfunction in the adult respiratory distress syndrome. Chest 1989;95:871–5.
9. Kenney EM, Rozanski EA, Rush JE, et al. Association between outcome and organ system dysfunction in dogs with sepsis: 114 cases (2003–2007). JAVMA 2010;236:83–7.
10. Sinanan M, Maier RV, Carrico CJ. Laparotomy for intraabdominal sepsis in patients in an intensive care unit. Arch Surg 1984;1:652–8.
11. Goris RJ, Boekhorsh TP, Nuytinic JK, et al. Multiple organ failure: generalized autodestructive inflammation? Arch Surg 1985;120:1109–15.
12. Marshall JC, Christou NV, Horn R, et al. The microbiology of multiple organ failure: the proximal gastrointestinal tract as an occult reservoir of pathogens. Arch Surg 1988;123:309–13.
13. Ahmed AJ, Kruse JA, Haupt MT, et al. Hemodynamic responses to gram-positive versus gram-negative sepsis in critically ill patients with and without circulatory shock. Crit Care Med 1991;19:1520–5.
14. Bone RC. The pathogenesis of sepsis. Ann Intern Med 1991;115:457–69.
15. Matuschak GM. Multiple organ system failure: clinical expression, pathogenesis, and therapy. In: Hall JB, Schmidt GA, Wood LDH, editors. Principles of critical care. New York: McGraw-Hill; 1998. p. 221.
16. Bone RC. Immunologic dissonance: a continuing evolution in our understanding of the systemic inflammatory response syndrome (SIRS) and the multiple organ dysfunction syndrome (MODS). Ann Intern Med 1996;125:680–7.
17. Moore FA, Moore EE. Evolving concepts in the pathogenesis of postinjury multiple organ failure. Surg Clin North Am 1995;75:257–77.
18. American College of Chest Physicians & Society of Critical Care Medicine Consensus Conference. Definitions for sepsis and organ failure, and guidelines for the use of innovative therapies in sepsis. Crit Care Med 1992;20:864–74.
19. Kirby R. Septic shock. In: Bonagura JD, editor. Current veterinary therapy XII. Philadelphia: W.B. Saunders Company; 1995. p. 139.
20. Peres Bota D, Melot C, Lopes Ferreira F, et al. The Multiple Organ Dysfunction Score (MODS) versus the Sequential Organ Dysfunction Failure Assessment (SOFA) score in outcome prediction. Intensive Care Med 2002;28:1619–24.
21. King LG, Wohl JS, Manning AM, et al. Evaluation of the survival prediction index as a model of risk stratification for clinical research in dogs admitted to intensive care units at four locations. Am J Vet Res 2001;62:948–54.

Respiratory Complications in Critical Illness of Small Animals

Vicki Lynne Campbell, DVM

KEYWORDS

- Acute respiratory distress syndrome • Acute lung injury
- Systemic inflammatory response syndrome • Sepsis
- Multiple organ dysfunction syndrome

The percentage of emergency patients with respiratory problems treated at veterinary emergency and critical care facilities is poorly defined. A study from the University of Pennsylvania indicated that 22% of patients undergoing laparotomy developed post-operative pulmonary complications,[1] including respiratory arrest, acute respiratory distress syndrome (ARDS), pneumonia, hypoventilation, and transient hypoxia.[1] Another study indicated that the chest is the most common region traumatized during blunt trauma, with blunt vehicular trauma accounting for 91.1% of those cases.[2] Thoracic trauma is common during polytrauma,[3] and pulmonary contusions are a common complication secondary to motor vehicle accidents.[4] Treatment of primary and secondary lung diseases is a significant element of emergency and critical care veterinary practice.

Regardless of whether an animal has a primary lung disease or develops a secondary lung disease during hospitalization, ARDS is a common sequela to the failing lung.[5] Acute lung injury (ALI) and ARDS are syndromes of pulmonary edema and inflammation of increasing severity.[6] There are many reported causes of ALI and ARDS in the literature. The primary causes include pneumonia, smoke inhalation, noncardiogenic edema, pulmonary contusions, lung lobe torsion, and hyperoxia.[1–8] ARDS is also caused by paraquat intoxication, pancreatitis, shock, sepsis, gastric/splenic torsion, babesiosis, rabies, bee envenomation, genetics, disseminated intravascular coagulation (DIC), and parvovirus (**Box 1**).[5–15]

In general, when injury happens, local inflammation occurs to rid the body of the damage and to allow repair. The body has natural antiinflammatory mechanisms that keep this proinflammatory stage in check and prevent it from going out of control.

Department of Clinical Sciences, Colorado State University, 300 West Drake Road, Fort Collins, CO 80523, USA
E-mail address: Vicki.Campbell@colostate.edu

Vet Clin Small Anim 41 (2011) 709–716
doi:10.1016/j.cvsm.2011.05.001   **vetsmall.theclinics.com**

Box 1
ACCP/SCCM consensus conference definitions of sepsis: the systemic inflammatory response syndrome (SIRS) to a documented infection

1. Severe sepsis/SIRS: Sepsis (SIRS) associated with organ dysfunction, hypoperfusion, or hypotension. Hypoperfusion and perfusion abnormalities may include, but are not limited to, lactic acidosis, oliguria, or an acute alteration in mental status.

2. Sepsis (SIRS)-induced hypotension: A systolic blood pressure less than 90 mm Hg or a reduction of more than 40 mm Hg from baseline in the absence of other causes of hypotension.

3. Septic shock/SIRS shock: A subset of severe sepsis (SIRS) and defined as sepsis (SIRS)-induced hypotension despite adequate fluid resuscitation along with the presence of perfusion abnormalities that may include, but are not limited to, lactic acidosis, oliguria, or an acute alteration in mental status.

4. Multiple organ dysfunction syndrome (MODS): Presence of altered organ function in an acutely ill patient such that homeostasis cannot be maintained without intervention.

Data from Bone RC, Balk RA, Cerra FB, et al. Definitions for sepsis and organ failure and guidelines for the use of innovative therapies in sepsis. The ACCP/SCCM Consensus Conference Committee. American College of Chest Physicians/Society of Critical Care Medicine. Chest 1992;101:1644–55.

When inflammation spirals out of control, the release of an overwhelming number of noxious substances may also cause damage to normal healthy tissue. Newly damaged tissue can induce more inflammation and a vicious cycle begins. Antiinflammatory systems in the body can be overwhelmed if the injury/inflammation sustains, new insults to the body (such as hypoxia, surgery) are present, or the immune system is compromised, such as with immune-mediated diseases. Activated neutrophils then travel to other parts of the body and accumulate in organs. In essence, the whole body starts to become inflamed and normal tissue is targeted and destroyed even at distant sites from the original injury. This out-of-control inflammation results in clinical signs that can be observed and has been given the term the SIRS.[16]

In patients with SIRS, the body responds in various ways to the excess release of cytokines, or hypercytokinemia, that is occurring in the body.[17] Most cytokines are released from activated monocytes, macrophages, and neutrophils. Thermoregulation, heart rate (HR), respiratory rate (RR), and white blood cell (WBC) counts frequently become altered. Pyrexia occurs because of the release of the cytokines interleukin-1 (IL-1) and IL-6. Tachycardia and tachypnea are stimulated by IL-1 and tumor necrosis factor (TNF)-α. Leukocytosis can occur because of granulocyte colony-stimulating factor, granulocyte monocyte stimulating factor, and IL-6. In addition, the circulating cytokines further activate neutrophils, which can result in end-organ damage.[16,17] As a result of the systemic responses that occur because of the excessive inflammation, SIRS can be defined when certain clinical criteria are met. In veterinary medicine, these clinical criteria for SIRS are based on an adaptation of human SIRS criteria.[18] To meet the SIRS criteria, dogs must have 2 or more of the following[19–21]:

Tachycardia (HR >120 bpm)
Tachypnea (RR >20 bpm)
Fever (>104.0°F) or hypothermia (<100.4°F)
Leukopenia (<5000 WBC/µL) or leukocytosis (>18,000 WBC/µL).

SIRS criteria for cats are slightly different than those for dogs. A cat must have 2 or more of the following to meet the SIRS criteria[22]:

Bradycardia (HR <140 bpm) or tachycardia (HR >225 bpm)
Tachypnea (RR >40 bpm)
Fever (>104.0°F) or hypothermia (<100.0°F)
Leukopenia (<5000 WBC/μL) or leukocytosis (>19,000 WBC/μL).

Some sources indicate that more than 5% or 10% of band neutrophils should also be considered as one of the criteria for SIRS.[19–23]

Because of the lack of sensitivity and specificity for the SIRS criteria, the human medical field has attempted to expand the classification scheme to better identify patients with sepsis. A newer classification scheme uses the old SIRS criteria and adds other physical parameters and biomarkers to identify patients with sepsis, known as PIRO (which stands for predisposition, insult, response, and organ dysfunction).[24,25] Predisposition may include genetic factors, age, concurrent conditions, or gender. Insult may include bacteria type, and location and extent of infection. Response uses biomarkers to look for evidence of excessive proinflammation, hypoinflammatory states, adrenal dysfunction, and coagulation abnormalities. Organ dysfunction may include renal failure and ARDS. Further studies in both human and veterinary medicine may determine the usefulness of the PIRO classification scheme.

It is important to be able to identify a patient who has SIRS because SIRS is frequently associated with sepsis. Sepsis is SIRS with infection.[18] In humans, severe sepsis is the third leading cause of death, with a mortality rate between 28% and 50% or greater.[25] If sepsis can be recognized in its early stages, there is a higher probability of treatment success. However, once sepsis leads to septic shock and multiple organ failure, the mortality rate increases dramatically. Therefore, it is necessary to recognize sepsis/SIRS in its early stages.

Sepsis has been grouped into 5 different stages by Bone.[17]

1. Establishment of infection: In this stage, infection sets up the initial inflammation and cytokine release. The body quickly begins proinflammatory mediator regulation with the compensatory antiinflammatory response to prevent excessive cytokine release and inflammation.
2. Preliminary systemic response: This is an indication that the infection has not been locally maintained. At this stage, fever is the most consistent systemic response.
3. Overwhelming systemic response: This is caused by excessive release of proinflammatory cytokines and mediators that produce the clinical syndrome of SIRS: tachycardia (or bradycardia in cats); tachypnea; pyrexia or hypothermia; and leukocytosis, leukopenia, or band neutrophilia.
4. Compensatory antiinflammatory reaction: The body tries to downregulate the proinflammatory mediators so that many of the signs of sepsis resolve. However, if this antiinflammatory reaction sustains for a long time, a syndrome called compensatory antiinflammatory response syndrome (CARS) occurs. CARS causes immune system paralysis and potentially allows the initial infection to spread or allows superinfection.
5. Immunomodulatory failure: This is the failure of the immune system to return to healthy homeostasis. In this stage, monocytes become deactivated and can no longer respond. Hence, the infection progresses, organ failure ensues, and death occurs.

In patients with sepsis, the development of MODS is a grave prognostic indicator. The greater the number of organs that develop dysfunction, the higher is the mortality rate. MODS, a multifactorial syndrome, is a result of insults and injuries secondary to SIRS or sepsis.[16]

One of the major effects of MODS is endothelial cell damage, secondary to the overwhelming release of proinflammatory cytokines. When endothelial cells are damaged, they are exposed to substances that activate the clotting cascade within the surrounding blood and tissue. Therefore, platelets aggregate, the secondary hemostatic pathways are stimulated, and clots form and then are ultimately broken down. When there is an overabundance of clotting, clotting factors are consumed. Once a significant number of clotting factors are depleted, spontaneous bleeding can occur. This imbalance of clotting and bleeding underlies DIC.[26] Microthrombosis from excessive clotting can lead to local tissue hypoxia and cellular death, leading to increases in inflammation.[26] Coagulation dysfunction (coagulation activation, abnormalities in fibrinolysis, and microcirculatory thrombosis), in addition to bacterial factors and excessive inflammatory mediators, promotes organ death and dysfunction.

ARDS and ALI are common sequelae to critical illness caused by SIRS, sepsis, and subsequent MODS.[5–7] In humans, the definition of ARDS includes acute onset of respiratory distress, hypoxemia, bilateral pulmonary infiltrates on radiographs, and pulmonary arterial wedge pressures less than 18 mm Hg. At sea level, an oxygen index or a partial pressure of dissolved arterial oxygen-to-inspired oxygen ratio (Pao_2:Fio_2) of 200 to 300 mm Hg is defined as ALI. Pao_2:Fio_2 less than 200 mm Hg is defined as ARDS.[27,28] The Dorothy Russell Havemeyer ALI and ARDS in Veterinary Medicine Consensus Group defined and published the first veterinary ALI and ARDS criteria in 2007.[6] Five criteria were proposed, the first 4 required and the fifth optional. These criteria are given in **Box 2**.[6]

The pathophysiology of ARDS is fairly well described.[5,29] ARDS begins with systemic or local pulmonary inflammation. Vasculitis then ensues, leading to increased pulmonary capillary permeability, causing protein-rich edema. The lungs then undergo exudative, proliferative, and fibrotic phases of ARDS. As lung inflammation increases, ensuing damage occurs. The macrophages and neutrophils release cytokines, leading to further damage and inflammation, specifically, TNF-α, IL-1, tumor growth factor-β, IL-6, platelet-activating factor, CXC chemokine ligand (IL-8), eicosanoids, and IL-10. This results in bilateral pulmonary infiltrates, hypoxemia, poor lung compliance, surfactant deficiency, pulmonary hypertension, vascular bed disruption/obstruction, hypoxic pulmonary vasoconstriction, and ultimately right-sided heart failure.

Monitoring and treatment are intensive in these patients, and experienced nursing care is critical. Frequently these patients need fluid therapy, pharmacologic blood pressure support, central venous pressure monitoring, direct arterial blood pressure monitoring, frequent blood gas analysis, blood products, and intravenous or enteral nutrition. Many of these animals are nonambulatory, so bladder/urinary care, colon care, passive range of motion, oral care, and prevention of pressure sores are important elements of treatment. Experienced personnel are needed to recognize dynamic changes in an animal's health status.

Many patients with ARDS require oxygen therapy and mechanical ventilation. Low tidal volumes paired with higher RRs are more lung protective, compared with high tidal volumes with lower RRs.[27,28,30,31] During mechanical ventilation, it is important to remain on the ideal portion of the pulmonary compliance curve, avoiding alveolar collapse and overdistention. This is achieved by providing positive end-expiratory pressure (PEEP), as well as avoiding high peak inspiratory pressures (PIPs). Prevention of oxygen toxicity by keeping the Fio_2 level less than 60% is also a lung protective strategy.

ARDS and ALI are best treated by addressing the underlying cause. The prognosis of these animals is usually poor, and the treatment, other than oxygen therapy and

---

Box 2
VetALI/VetARDS

1. Acute onset (<72 hours) of tachypnea and labored breathing at rest

2. Known risk factors

   a. Inflammation

   b. Infection

   c. Multiple transfusion

   d. Sepsis

   e. Smoke inhalation

   f. Near drowning

   g. SIRS

   h. Aspiration

   i. Severe trauma

   j. Drugs and toxin

3. Evidence of pulmonary capillary leak without increased pulmonary capillary pressure (pulmonary artery occlusion pressure <18 mm Hg) or no clinical or diagnostic evidence of left-sided heart failure (because of 1 or more of the following):

   a. Bilateral/diffuse infiltrates on thoracic radiographs (more than 1 quadrant/lobe)

   b. Bilateral dependent density gradient on computed tomography

   c. Proteinaceous fluid within the conducting airways

   d. Increased extravascular lung water

4. Evidence of inefficient gas exchange (1 or more of the following):

   a. Hypoxemia without PEEP or continuous positive airway pressure and known Fio_2: Pao_2:Fio_2 ratio <300 mm Hg for VetALI; Pao_2:Fio_2 ratio <200 mm Hg for VetARDS; increased A-a gradient; venous admixture (noncardiac shunt)

   b. Increased dead space ventilation

5. Evidence of diffuse pulmonary inflammation

   a. Transtracheal wash/bronchoalveolar lavage sample neutrophilia

   b. Molecular imaging (positron emission tomography)

From Wilkins PA, Otto CM, Baumgardner JE, et al. Acute lung injury and acute respiratory distress syndromes in veterinary medicine: consensus definitions: the Dorothy Russell Havemeyer Working Group on ALI and ARDS in Veterinary Medicine. JVECCS 2007;17(4):333–9; with permission.

---

mechanical ventilation, is controversial. The human medical literature has indicated that conservative fluid management, compared with liberal fluid management, in patients with ALI leads to more ventilator-free days and more intensive care unit–free days and does not lead to an increased incidence of renal dysfunction.[32] Several human studies have indicated that a combination of furosemide and a colloid (usually albumin) improves oxygenation, hemodynamics, and fluid balance in ALI, compared with furosemide alone or placebo, especially in patients who are hypoproteinemic.[33–35] Constant rate infusions of furosemide may be more effective than bolus dosing,[36] and the author has used 0.1 to 0.2 mg/kg/h of furosemide in combination with albumin in patients with ARDS and ALI with some success.

Additional nonventilatory treatments of ALI and ARDS that have been used in human medicine include surfactant, inhaled nitric oxide, corticosteroids, antifungal agents, and phosphodiesterase inhibitors.[37] None of these treatments have been shown to have a mortality benefit.[37]

Phosphodiesterase 5 inhibitors (P-5Is) are frequently used to help counteract pulmonary hypertension, which can be a secondary complication in ARDS and ALI. The most commonly used phosphodiesterase inhibitor for this purpose in veterinary medicine is sildenafil. To the author's knowledge, there have been no veterinary research studies using P-5Is in patients with ARDS or ALI. P-5Is have had no mortality benefit in human patients with ARDS and ALI.[37] The veterinary literature indicates that sildenafil is not specific to the pulmonary circulation.[38] There is conflicting evidence that sildenafil decreases pulmonary hypertension, although most studies have concluded that it improves clinical signs and quality of life in animals.[39–41] In a canine study, the median dose of sildenafil was 1.9 mg/kg and the median pulmonary arterial pressure decreased by 16.5 mm Hg with treatment and most clinical signs resolved.[41] If pulmonary hypertension is present, it may be worth pursuing this treatment.

Future avenues of nonventilator therapeutic study on ARDS/ALI in human medicine include inhaled beta-agonist therapy, which may decrease lung water and inflammation; granulocyte-macrophage colony-stimulating factor, which maintains alveolar macrophage function and prevents alveolar epithelial apoptosis; and activated protein C, which may reduce lung inflammation and inhibits coagulation.[37]

Indications of beneficial response to treatment include gradual improvement in arterial blood gases, improved oxygen index, decreased amount of PEEP needed to maintain oxygenation on the ventilator, decreased PIPs indicating improved compliance, decreased work of breathing, and improved lung auscultation.

In summary, ARDS is a frequent sequela to sepsis, SIRS, and DIC and is frequently the pulmonary manifestation of MODS. ARDS, ALI, SIRS, sepsis, and MODS are serious syndromes with grave consequences. Understanding the pathophysiology and consequences of these syndromes is imperative to early recognition.

REFERENCES

1. Alwood AJ, Brainard BM, LaFond E, et al. Postoperative pulmonary complications in dogs undergoing laparotomy: frequency, characterization and disease-related risk factors. JVECCS 2006;16(3):176–83.
2. Simpson SA, Syring R, Otto CM. Severe blunt trauma in dogs: 235 cases (1997–2003). JVECCS 2009;19(6):588–602.
3. Selcer BA, Buttrick M, Barstad R, et al. The incidence of thoracic trauma in dogs with skeletal injury. J Small Anim Pract 1987;28(1):21–7.
4. Powell LL, Rozanski EA, Tidwell AS, et al. A retrospective analysis of pulmonary contusion secondary to motor vehicular accidents in 143 dogs: 1994–1997. J Vet Emerg Crit Care 1999;9(3):127–36.
5. Parent C, King L, Walker L, et al. Clinical and clinicopathologic finding in dogs with acute respiratory distress syndrome: 19 cases (1985–1993). J Am Med Vet Assoc 1996;208(9):1419–27.
6. Wilkins PA, Otto CM, Baumgardner JE, et al. Acute lung injury and acute respiratory distress syndromes in veterinary medicine: consensus definitions: the Dorothy Russell Havemeyer Working Group on ALI and ARDS in Veterinary Medicine. JVECCS 2007;17(4):333–9.

7. Parent C, King L, VanWinkle TJ, et al. Respiratory function and treatment in dogs with acute respiratory distress syndrome: 19 cases (1983–1993). J Am Med Vet Assoc 1996;208(9):1428–33.

8. DeClue AE, Cohn LA. Acute respiratory distress syndrome in dogs and cats: a review of clinical findings and pathophysiology. JVECCS 2007;17(4):340–7.

9. Darke P, Gibbs C, Kelly D, et al. Acute respiratory distress in the dog associated with paraquat poisoning. Vet Rec 1977;100(14):275–7.

10. Hsu YH, Chen HI. Acute respiratory distress syndrome associated with rabies. Pathology 2008;40(6):647–50.

11. Walker T, Tidwell AS, Rozanski EA, et al. Imaging diagnosis: acute lung injury following massive bee envenomation in a dog. Vet Radiol Ultrasound 2005; 56(4):300–3.

12. Syrja P, Saari S, Rajamaki M, et al. Pulmonary histopathology in Dalmatians with familial acute respiratory distress syndrome (ARDS). J Comp Pathol 2009;141(4): 254–9.

13. Lopez A, Lane I, Hanna P. Adult respiratory distress syndrome in a dog with necrotizing pancreatitis. Can Vet J 1995;36:240–1.

14. Mohr A, Lobetti R, Lugt J. Acute pancreatitis: a newly recognized potential complication of canine babesiosis. J S Afr Vet Assc 2000;71:232–9.

15. Neath P, Brockman D, King L. Lung lobe torsion in dogs: 22 cases (1981–1999). J Am Med Vet Assoc 2000;217:1041–4.

16. Davies MG, Hagen PO. Systemic inflammatory response syndrome. Br J Surg 1997;84:920–35.

17. Bone RC. Toward a theory regarding the pathogenesis of the systemic inflammatory response system: what we do and do not know about cytokine regulation. Crit Care Med 1996;24:163–72.

18. Bone RC, Balk RA, Cerra FB, et al. Definitions for sepsis and organ failure and guidelines for the use of innovative therapies in sepsis. The ACCP/SCCM Consensus Conference Committee. American College of Chest Physicians/ Society of Critical Care Medicine. Chest 1992;101:1644–55.

19. Haptman JG, Walshaw R, Olivier NB. Evaluation of the sensitivity and specificity of diagnostic criteria for sepsis in dogs. Vet Surg 1997;26:393–7.

20. Hardie EM. Life-threatening bacterial infection. Compend Contin Educ Pract Vet 1995;17:763–77.

21. Purvis D, Kirby R. Systemic inflammatory response syndrome: septic shock. Vet Clin North Am 1994;24:1225–47.

22. Brady C, Otto C, Van Winkle T, et al. Severe sepsis in cats: a retrospective study of 29 cases (1986–1998). JAVMA 2000;217:531–5.

23. Okano S, Yoshida M, Fukushima, et al. Usefulness of systemic inflammatory response syndrome criteria as an index for prognosis judgment. Vet Rec 2002; 150:245–6.

24. Balk RA, Ely WE, Goyette RE. Sepsis handbook. 2nd edition. Nashville (TN): Thomson Advanced Therapeutics Communications and Vanderbilt University School of Medicine; 2004.

25. Dellinger RP, Carlet JM, Masur H, et al. Surviving sepsis campaign guidelines for management of severe sepsis and septic shock. Crit Care Med 2004;32:858–73.

26. Hopper K, Bateman S. An updated view of hemostasis: mechanisms of hemostatic dysfunction associated with sepsis. JVECCS 2005;15(2):83–91.

27. Bernard G, Artigas A, Brigham K, et al. The American-European Consensus Conference on ARDS. Definitions, mechanisms, relevant outcomes, and clinical trial coordination. Am J Respir Crit Care Med 1994;149:818–24.

28. Artigas A, Bernard GR, Arlet J, et al. The American-European consensus conference on ARDS, part 2: ventilator, pharmacologic, supportive therapy, study design strategies and issues related to recovery and remodeling. Am J Respir Crit Care Med 1998;157:1332–47.
29. Tamashefski J. Pulmonary pathology of the adult respiratory distress syndrome. Clin Chest Med 1990;11:593–619.
30. Gillete MA, Hess DR. Ventilator-induced lung injury and the evolution of lung-protective strategies in acute respiratory distress syndrome. Respir Care 2001; 46(2):130–48.
31. Mueller ER. Suggested strategies for ventilator management of veterinary patients with acute respiratory distress syndrome. JVECCS 2001;11(3):191–8.
32. Acute Respiratory Distress Syndrome Network. Comparison of two fluid-management strategies in acute lung injury. N Engl J Med 2006;354:2564–75.
33. Martin GS. Fluid balance and colloid osmotic pressure in acute respiratory failure: emerging clinical evidence. Crit Care 2000;4(Suppl 2):S21–5.
34. Martin GS, Mangialardi RJ, Wheeler AP, et al. Albumin and furosemide therapy in hypoproteinemic patients with acute lung injury. Crit Care Med 2002;30:2175–82.
35. Martin GS, Moss M, Wheeler AP, et al. A randomized controlled trial of furosemide with or without albumin in hypoproteinemic patients with acute lung injury. Crit Care Med 2005;33:1681–7.
36. Martin SJ, Danziger LH. Continuous infusion of loop diuretics in the critically ill: a review of the literature. Crit Care Med 1994;22:1323–9.
37. Calfee CS, Matthay MA. Nonventilatory treatments for acute lung injury and ARDS. Chest 2007;131:913–20.
38. Fesler P, Pagnamenta A, Rondelet B, et al. Effects of sildenafil on hypoxic pulmonary vascular function in dogs. J Appl Physiol 2006;101(4):1085–90.
39. Brown AJ, Davison E, Sleeper MM. Clinical efficacy of sildenafil in treatment of pulmonary arterial hypertension in dogs. J Vet Intern Med 2010;24(4):850–4.
40. Kellum HB, Stepien RL. Sildenafil citrate therapy in 22 dogs with pulmonary hypertension. J Vet Intern Med 2007;21(6):1258–64.
41. Bach JF, Rozanski EA, MacGregor J, et al. Retrospective evaluation of sildenafil citrate as a therapy for pulmonary hypertension in dogs. J Vet Intern Med 2006; 20(5):1132–5.

Cardiovascular Dysfunction in Sepsis and Critical Illness

Barret J. Bulmer, DVM, MS

KEYWORDS

• Echocardiography • SIRS • Systolic dysfunction
• Myocardial depressant factor

Sepsis, trauma, major surgery, and other noninfectious conditions including autoimmune disease, vasculitis, thromboembolism, and burns can illicit severe, and often uncontrolled, activation of the immune system and mediator cells. Complex and still poorly understood cellular interactions can commence provoking a systemic inflammatory response syndrome (SIRS) with clinical features of tachypnea, hypothermia or hyperthermia, leukocytosis, myocardial dysfunction and hypotension that is hyporesponsive to pressors. Recent evidence also suggests that, as sepsis persists, there is a shift toward an immunosuppressive state.[1] Although there are numerous causes for induction of SIRS, all of which may share common pathways, sepsis is the most thoroughly investigated, principally because it is a leading cause of death in critically ill patients. Sepsis accounts annually for at least 210,000 human deaths in the United States, with a reported mortality as high as 30% to 50%.[1] More striking is that in the 40% of patients who experience myocardial dysfunction as a complication of sepsis, the mortality rises to 70% to 90%.[2] Data for small numbers of cases suggest that myocardial dysfunction accompanies sepsis and SIRS in dogs and cats. However, because the data from small animals are minimal, the following discussion primarily focuses on mechanisms of myocardial dysfunction and potential therapeutic opportunities in humans.

CARDIAC PERFORMANCE IN SEPTIC SHOCK
Humans

Initial studies in humans suggested that the hallmark cardiovascular pattern in septic shock was a low-output, hypodynamic circulation that contributed to cold and clammy skin and a thready pulse with hypotension. However, these studies used central venous pressure as a measure of ventricular preload, as opposed to

This work is unsupported by grant funding.
The author has nothing to disclose.
Department of Clinical Sciences, Cummings School of Veterinary Medicine at Tufts University, 200 Westboro Road, North Grafton, MA 01536, USA
E-mail address: Barret.Bulmer@tufts.edu

Vet Clin Small Anim 41 (2011) 717–726
doi:10.1016/j.cvsm.2011.04.003   vetsmall.theclinics.com
0195-5616/11/$ – see front matter © 2011 Elsevier Inc. All rights reserved.

pulmonary capillary wedge pressure, and it is likely that many of the patients had inadequate left ventricular filling.[3] Later studies performed under adequate volume resuscitation found that hypotension was more likely the product of profound reduction in systemic vascular resistance, and the more typical cardiovascular pattern in septic patients was high cardiac output with an increased cardiac index.[4]

As advances in the use of radionuclide-gated blood pool scanning, catheter-derived thermodilution techniques, and echocardiography became commonplace, more accurate measures of ventricular performance and volume could be obtained. These techniques found that, despite normal cardiac output, patients with septic shock did experience myocardial dysfunction. The characteristic cardiac changes seen in survivors of septic shock consist of decreased left ventricular ejection fraction and increased end-diastolic and end-systolic volume indices within 24 hours of the onset of septic shock.[5] Patients experience a reduced post–fluid resuscitation left ventricular ejection fraction, ventricular dilation, and flattening of the Frank-Starling relationship compared with critically ill, nonseptic controls.[6] The myocardial depression is reversible in survivors, with ventricular size and function returning to normal within 7 to 10 days after the episode of septic shock.[5] Nonsurvivors lack the characteristic left ventricular dilation and decreased ejection fraction.[5] It is hypothesized that ventricular dilation may be a compensatory response; hence, in its absence, there is higher mortality.[3] Advances in echocardiographic techniques are also providing insight into additional factors, including diastolic dysfunction and myocardial compliance abnormalities that may contribute further to myocardial dysfunction in sepsis.

Dogs

Although canine models have provided valuable information into the mechanisms of cardiovascular dysfunction in sepsis and SIRS for decades, there is little information regarding its prevalence or prognosis with naturally occurring disease. Limitations for assessment and investigation of myocardial performance in dogs with critical illness include infrequent monitoring of cardiac output or pulmonary capillary wedge pressure via Swan-Ganz catheterization and difficulty assessing the load-independent function of the heart.

In 2006, Nelson and Thompson[7] reported a retrospective study of 16 dogs with left ventricular dysfunction associated with severe systemic illness. In this population, critical illness was defined as metabolic derangements that required intensive care to sustain life, and left ventricular systolic dysfunction was defined as a fractional shortening of less than 26% and/or an ejection fraction of less than 46%. Dogs with a left ventricular preejection period/ejection time ratio of more than 0.4 were also considered to have systolic dysfunction. The 2 most common diseases identified producing critical illness with left ventricular systolic dysfunction were sepsis (n = 5) and cancer (n = 5).[7] Twelve of the 16 dogs (75%) died or were euthanized within 15 days of hospital admission, with an average time until death of 3.6 days. Treatment regimens for the dogs varied considerably so comparison between survivors and nonsurvivors was not performed. The 4 dogs that were discharged had follow-up of 20 days, 3.5 months, 4 months, and 2 years. Longitudinal echocardiographic data were available only for a boxer dog with immune-mediated polyarthropathy, anemia, and hyperglobulinemia that was still alive 2 years after hospitalization. The fractional shortening had risen from 21% at the time of hospitalization to 34% 2 years later, suggesting reversible myocardial depression. Dickinson and colleagues[8] subsequently reported reversible myocardial depression in a 5-month-old Rhodesian ridgeback with sepsis. At the time of hospitalization, the dog displayed an enlarged end-systolic volume index at 41 mL/m^2 that had decreased to 16.5 mL/m^2 3 months later. Recently,

Kenney and colleagues[9] reported a large-scale study of the association between outcome and organ system dysfunction in dogs with sepsis secondary to gastrointestinal tract leakage. Cardiovascular dysfunction was defined as hypotension sufficiently severe to require vasopressor treatment after surgery. Sepsis-induced myocardial depression was not evaluated via echocardiography. Twenty (17.5%) of the 114 dogs met the criteria for cardiovascular dysfunction and only 2 of the 20 survived to discharge from the hospital. When the results of these studies are taken in total, it suggests that myocardial dysfunction from sepsis occurs in dogs.

PROPOSED MECHANISMS OF SEPSIS-INDUCED MYOCARDIAL DYSFUNCTION

The first proposed theory for septic myocardial depression that was touted for decades was hypotension and hypoperfusion leading to myocardial dysfunction via global ischemia.[10] Animal models of endotoxic shock repeatedly showed global myocardial hypoperfusion; however, it was ultimately determined that this model, which used large lethal doses of intravenous endotoxin or live bacteria, did not produce a cardiovascular profile representative of what is seen in humans. Recent studies have identified that septic patients have high coronary blood flow and diminished coronary artery–coronary sinus oxygen difference.[4] Accordingly, a second major theory arose with origins that can be traced back to the study by Wiggers[11] wherein he postulated a circulating myocardial depressant factor. Waisbren[12] was the first to report myocardial dysfunction in patients with sepsis, and subsequent experimental studies were able to confirm the suspected myocardial depressant factor in sepsis.[13] The study by Parrillo and colleagues,[14] wherein patients' septic serum generated concentration-dependent depression of in vitro myocyte contractility, was the first study to corroborate the long-suspected link between septic shock and a circulating myocardial depressant factor.

Attempts to identify a specific myocardial depressant substance (MDS) continued after the study by Parrillo and colleagues,[14] and hemofiltration studies found that the stimulating factor in patients' sera was greater than 10 kDa, heat labile, and water soluble, suggesting a protein or polypeptide.[15] Lipopolysaccharide (LPS) was postulated to represent the MDS because its infusion in animals and humans produced the hyperdynamic, hypotensive state seen in naturally occurring septic shock.[15] Although endotoxin was sufficient to produce septic shock, it was unlikely to explain the complete mechanism in itself. Experimental studies found that gram-positive bacteria produced the same pattern of cardiovascular changes as those invoked by endotoxin.[3] Furthermore, the prolonged time course for myocardial depression was not supportive of LPS as the sole substance, and many patients that were culture negative or had no detectable levels of endotoxemia still manifest the typical cardiovascular profile of patients with septic shock. These findings suggested that endotoxin, and likely several other triggers of myocardial dysfunction in sepsis, SIRS, and critical illness, share a common pathway wherein they contribute to activation of an endogenous cascade of local and systemic inflammatory mediators. If the inflammatory response is intense, it may ultimately lead to shock and potentially myocardial depression. The cascade from presumed immunodetection of LPS (and other triggers of sepsis and SIRS) to myocardial dysfunction has been extensively studied and remains incompletely elucidated. However, considerable progress has been made since the landmark study by Wiggers,[11] and many emerging concepts have been described in the past decade that provide opportunities for understanding the pathogenesis of sepsis-induced myocardial depression and provide possible opportunities to mitigate this process.

TOLL-LIKE RECEPTORS AND INNATE IMMUNITY

In 1997, a human homolog of the *Drosophila* Toll protein was identified that serves as a nonclonal receptor of the innate immune system.[16] Transfection of an active mutant Toll-like receptor (TLR) into human cell lines was able to induce activation of NF-κB and promote gene expression for numerous cytokines.[16] To date, 11 human TLRs have been identified representing germline-encoded receptor proteins that recognize specific patterns shared by groups of pathogens, but not the host.[17] TLR2 is a plasma membrane–localized receptor that recognizes specific cell wall components of gram-positive bacteria, gram-negative bacteria, mycobacteria, fungi, parasites, and viruses, whereas TLR4 binds to specific components of LPS, pneumolysin of *streptococcus* pneumonia, the F-protein of respiratory syncytial virus, and an envelope glycoprotein encoded by mouse mammary tumor virus.[17–19] Although it is hypothesized that the TLRs serve as pattern recognition receptors that are able to differentiate host from pathogen, studies have identified ligand recognition of heat shock proteins and extracellular domain A in fibronectin via TLR4.[17,19] Therefore, even in the absence of pathogens, tissue destruction may stimulate the innate immune system and downstream inflammatory cascade via release of fragments of hyaluronan and fibronectin and subsequent binding to TLR2 or TLR4.[17] Additional currently unknown ligands may link TLRs and myocardial depression in sepsis, SIRS, and critical illness that are unrelated to LPS. However, most research to date has focused on the mechanisms wherein endotoxin produces myocardial dysfunction.

TLR4 is profoundly important for LPS-mediated effects, as shown by TLR4-deficient mice being completely resistant to endotoxic shock exhibiting no early neutropenia, no leukocyte infiltration into organs, and no detectable mortality.[20] Immune cell detection of LPS is hypothesized to initiate myocyte dysfunction in the first few hours of endotoxemia as circulating leukocytes rapidly infiltrate cardiac tissue during inflammation. The finding that hearts perfused with leukocyte-depleted, endotoxemic blood displayed normal pressure generation and those receiving unfiltered blood displayed impaired left ventricular pressure generation[21] led to more detailed studies of LPS-induced myocyte impairment. In 2004, Tavener and Kubes[22] reported that TLR4-positive bone marrow–derived leukocytes, as opposed to direct LPS-mediated toxicity to myocardial cells, were responsible for acute (within 4 hours) LPS-induced myocyte dysfunction.[20] Subsequent studies identified that neutrophil-deficient or mast cell–deficient mice exposed to LPS had similar reductions in shortening of ventricular myocytes compared with controls, suggesting that neither cell type alone contributes to myocardial depression.[22] Macrophage-deficient mice exposed to LPS displayed partial reduction of myocyte impairment, and mice that were macrophage and neutrophil deficient exposed to LPS had complete restoration of myocyte shortening.[22] LPS-mediated signal transduction in tissues other than leukocytes (eg, cardiac myocytes and microvascular endothelial cells) must also play a role in longer-term (18 hours after LPS injection) modulation of cardiac dysfunction because inactivation of marrow-derived TLR4 function alone is incapable of protecting against endotoxin-triggered contractile dysfunction.[23] TLR2 has been implicated in *Staphylococcus aureus*[24] and polymicrobial sepsis–induced[25] myocardial dysfunction, and bacterial DNA has been shown to induce myocardial inflammation and reduced cardiac contractility via TLR9.[26] Whether other antigenic stimuli or host-recognized ligands contribute to myocardial dysfunction in sepsis, SIRS, and multiorgan dysfunction syndrome (MODS) is uncertain, but is hypothesized.

CASCADE OF EVENTS FROM TRIGGER TO MYOCARDIAL DYSFUNCTION

Detection of LPS begins with recognition and binding by the acute-phase protein, LPS-binding protein (LBP).[27] LBP aids docking of LPS to CD14, which was once believed to be the LPS receptor, but now seems more likely to present and enable binding of LPS to an MD-2/TLR4 complex. MD-2 serves as an essential extracellular adaptor protein and, when complexed with LPS and TLR4, initiates signal transduction.[28,29] The intracellular signaling motif is similar to that for interleukin (IL)-1 and IL-18 receptors and is now termed the Toll–IL-1 receptor (TIR) homology domain.[17] There are numerous and variable cytoplasmic adaptor molecules, including myeloid differentiation primary response protein (MyD88), TIR domain–containing adaptor protein (TIRAP, also known as MyD88 adaptor like protein or Mal), TIR domain–containing adaptor-inducing interferon β (TRIF), and TRIF-related adaptor molecule (TRAM). Tissue-specific expression of TLRs and adaptors enables immune triggering with some degree of specificity and tailored immune responses for different pathogen-associated molecular patterns in a cell-dependent manner.[17] This variable expression likely contributes to the wide array of disease processes, including sepsis, atherosclerosis, liver injury, ischemia/reperfusion injury, kidney disease, inflammatory bowel disease, pulmonary disease, and acute doxorubicin toxicity that have been linked to TLRs.[19,30,31] LPS effector responses following TLR4 binding seem to be divided into an early MyD88-dependent response and a delayed MyD88-independent response.[27]

Binding of LPS to the MD-2/TLR4 receptor complex induces homodimerization and recruitment of MyD88 and TIRAP to the receptor complex.[27] MyD88 subsequently recruits members of the IL-1 receptor-associated kinase (IRAK) family, IRAK1 and IRAK4, which phosphorylate and activate tumor necrosis factor (TNF) receptor-associated factor 6 (TRAF6).[32] TRAF6 associates with TAK1-binding protein 2 (TAB2) and activates transforming growth factor β–activated kinase (TAK-1) and its constituent adaptor protein TAB1. TAK-1 activates the p38 and c-jun N-terminal kinase (JNK) MAPK pathways and begins the activation of NFκB by triggering assembly of a high-molecular-weight protein complex composed of inhibitory-binding protein κB kinase (IKK)α and IKKβ together with IKKγ. Ubiquitination and degradation of this protein complex occurs following phosphorylation of a set of inhibitory-binding proteins κB (IκB), ultimately releasing NFκB and enabling its translocation into the nucleus.[27] Gene transcription of proinflammatory cytokines subsequently occurs with elaboration of proinflammatory cytokines including, but not limited to, TNF-α, IL-1, IL-6, IL-18, and COX2.[27,32] Delayed nuclear translocation of NFκB and phosphorylation of interferon regulatory factor 3 (IRF3) to produce interferon β in response to LPS binding to TLR4 occurs via MyD88-independent pathways using the adaptor proteins TRIF and TRAM.[27]

Numerous molecular mechanisms have been hypothesized to link induction of cytokine production with impaired myocardial function, and studies suggest that there could be different factors producing early and delayed dysfunction. Platelet-activating factor (PAF) has been reported to directly decrease myocardial contractility via a specific, high-affinity cardiac PAF receptor.[33] PAF-mediated decreases in beating amplitude, velocity of contraction, and velocity of relaxation in cardiomyocytes seems at least partially explained via induction of the phosphoinositide pathway with resulting increases in inositol 1,4,5-triphosphate (IP3) and 1,2-diacylglycerol (DAG). Subsequent protein kinase C (PKC) activation results in negative inotropic responses.[33] TNF-α–mediated alterations in calcium homeostasis, potentially via sarcoplasmic reticular dysfunction, has been hypothesized as a contributing factor.[34] Heard and colleagues[35] also found increased PKC concentrations and a suspected alteration of calcium release from the sarcoplasmic reticulum in LPS-induced myocardial depression in guinea pigs, although PKC inhibition was unable to ameliorate the adverse cardiac effects of LPS. Further alterations in calcium homeostasis and ion flux provoking negative inotropism have been postulated via induction of the neutral sphingomyelinase pathway by TNF-α.[36,37] Studies suggest that downregulation of the L-type calcium channels[38,39] and decreased myocardial filament sensitivity to the prevailing calcium concentration[40,41] may also contribute to myocardial dysfunction in endotoxemia. TNF-α is suggested to induce a defective contractile response to catecholamines, so-called adrenergic uncoupling, as a result of severely impaired generation of cAMP.[6] Prostanoids, including thromboxane and prostacyclin, may contribute to impaired cardiac function by altering coronary autoregulation and coronary endothelial function and promoting intracoronary leukocyte activation,[4] whereas LPS-induced upregulation of endothelin-1 (ET-1) may produce dysregulation of systemic and regional vascular tone and itself may trigger increased inflammatory cytokines and nitric oxide (NO).[42] Adhesion molecules, including intercellular adhesion molecule-1 (ICAM-1), may also serve as myocardial depressant substrates through both neutrophil-dependent and neutrophil-independent mechanisms.[43–45]

Potentially the most investigated mechanism contributing to myocardial dysfunction in sepsis has been the role of NO and whether it serves deleterious or beneficial effects. NO-mediated effects could theoretically be helpful via correction of endothelial dysfunction and promotion of coronary vasodilation, improvement of left ventricular relaxation, inhibition of platelet and neutrophil adhesion and activation, and inhibition of cardiac oxygen consumption. However, NO also mediates detrimental cardiovascular effects via alterations of protein kinase A and, therefore, the L-type calcium channel, decreased myofibrillar response to calcium, and decreased cAMP via phosphodiesterase.[15] NO also stimulates macrophages and the respiratory burst of neutrophils, inhibits mitochondrial function, and potentially forms a major link in the myocardial depression observed in sepsis and SIRS via production of peroxynitrite when it combines with superoxide.[15] Peroxynitrite contributes to apoptosis and promotes tissue injury via lipid peroxidation, depletion of antioxidant reserves, oxidation/nitration of proteins including mitochondrial proteins, and induction of DNA damage, thereby activating poly(ADP)-ribose polymerase (PARP).[46] It further contributes to circulatory shock by promoting peripheral vascular failure, vascular endothelial dysfunction, myocardial depression, systemic inflammation, tissue leukocyte sequestration, and gut mucosal barrier failure.[46] A recent study suggests that increased NO production via the inducible form of nitric oxide synthase may contribute to extensive fetal-like shifts in gene expression with reductions in contractile protein expression, growth related genes, and energy-yielding genes.[47]

ADDITIONAL CONTRIBUTING FACTORS LEADING TO POOR OUTCOME

Myocardial depression is not the only alteration that contributes to higher mortality and a less favorable prognosis in patients with sepsis and SIRS experiencing cardiac dysfunction. Assessment of heart rate variability suggests cardiac autonomic dysfunction, with altered sympathetic and vagal regulation of heart function.[48] Reduced heart rate variability and an increased heart rate have both been identified as unfavorable prognostic factors in sepsis. Detrimental cardiac effects of sympathetic overstimulation may include tachycardia and impaired diastolic function, tachyarrhythmias, myocardial ischemia, stunning, apoptosis, and myocardial necrosis.[49] Autonomic impairment identified experimentally following endotoxin exposure could be related to alterations within the brain, the autonomic nervous system, or the pacemaker cell itself.[48] Studies have identified that endotoxin-induced alterations of heart rate variability are mediated, at least in part, by direct interaction with the cardiac pacemaker cells. Endotoxin directly targets the pacemaker funny current, I_f, which is normally the result of ion movement across the hyperpolarization-activated cyclic nucleotide-gated (HCN) channel. Endotoxin significantly impairs human atrial I_f via channel suppression at membrane potentials positive to -80 mV and by slowing down current activation at most tested potentials.[50] Computer simulations suggest that the channel alteration would diminish the ability of I_f to change cycle length in response to varying autonomic stimuli reducing heart rate variability and presumably slowing heart rate.[50] However, patients with sepsis and SIRS usually have an inappropriately high heart rate. Contributing factors enabling the heart rate to override endotoxin-reduced I_f activity include attenuated vagal tone, endogenous catecholamine release, in some instances exogenous catecholamine treatment, and a surprising endotoxin-mediated sensitization of I_f/HCN channels to β_1-adrenergic catecholamines.[48,50] HCN channels are also expressed in the brain, so the role of endotoxin on autonomic dysfunction may extend well beyond the heart.[48]

THERAPEUTIC POTENTIALS

General treatment of sepsis and SIRS usually entails targeting the underlying cause, ensuring adequate fluid resuscitation, and attempts to correct hypotension and maintain end-organ perfusion via the use of positive inotropes and vasopressors. Early (treatment during the initial 6 hours of presentation) goal-directed therapy to optimize preload, afterload, arterial oxygen content, and contractility, with balancing of systemic oxygen delivery and consumption, has significantly improved survival in humans with severe sepsis and septic shock.[51] These goals and the invasive method used to accomplish several of the endpoints, are not universally accepted in humans,[52] and similar studies have not been reported in dogs and cats. Nonetheless, maintenance of vascular tone and cardiac contractility in adequately volume-resuscitated patients may provide benefit and prevent deterioration along the continuum of self-limiting SIRS to severe sepsis and septic shock. Currently, vasopressor selection is often dictated by clinician preference and response to therapy. Hypotension related to reduced cardiac contractility may best be managed by constant rate infusions of dobutamine or dopamine, whereas α-agonists like norepinephrine may be superior for management of hypotension secondary to loss of systemic vascular resistance.[53] There may be additional emerging roles for vasopressin and vasopressin receptor antagonists in the management of refractory hypotension.[54]

Based on the complex mechanisms wherein sepsis, SIRS, and MODS are hypothesized to contribute to myocardial dysfunction and ultimately death, there are numerous potential novel targets that may further enhance outcome as opposed to general treatment alone. Many specific treatment strategies have seemed promising in the laboratory setting only to be met with disappointment in the clinical setting, likely indicating that a single mechanism alone does not account for the clinical scenario of myocardial dysfunction and its contribution to mortality. Outcome for the numerous specific treatment strategies that have been attempted is outside of the scope of this article, but they have included anti-LPS antibodies, anti–TNF-α antibodies, free radical scavengers, corticosteroids, nonsteroidal anti-inflammatory drugs, and nitric oxide inhibition.[15] These strategies continue to be analyzed[55] and modified. Statins, β-blockers, and angiotensin-converting enzyme inhibitors are being investigated for potential improvement in outcome via normalization of autonomic function.[48] In addition, the recent expansion of research into the immunoregulation of sepsis has led to numerous potential targets for mitigating TLR induction of myocardial depression via anti-TLR4 and TLR4–MD-2 complex antibodies, eritoran, resatorvid, chloroquine, ketamine, nicotine, opioids, statins, and vitamin D3 and its analogues.[56]

REFERENCES

1. Hotchkiss RS, Karl IE. The pathophysiology and treatment of sepsis. N Engl J Med 2003;348(2):138–50.
2. Parrillo JE, Parker MM, Natanson C, et al. Septic shock in humans. Advances in the understanding of pathogenesis, cardiovascular dysfunction, and therapy. Ann Intern Med 1990;113(3):227–42.
3. Snell RJ, Parrillo JE. Cardiovascular dysfunction in septic shock. Chest 1991; 99(4):1000–9.
4. Merx MW, Weber C. Sepsis and the heart. Circulation 2007;116(7):793–802.
5. Parker MM, Shelhamer JH, Bacharach SL, et al. Profound but reversible myocardial depression in patients with septic shock. Ann Intern Med 1984;100(4):483–90.
6. Kumar A, Haery C, Parrillo JE. Myocardial dysfunction in septic shock. Crit Care Clin 2000;16(2):251–87.
7. Nelson OL, Thompson PA. Cardiovascular dysfunction in dogs associated with critical illnesses. J Am Anim Hosp Assoc 2006;42(5):344–9.
8. Dickinson AE, Rozanski EA, Rush JE. Reversible myocardial depression associated with sepsis in a dog. J Vet Intern Med 2007;21(5):1117–20.
9. Kenney EM, Rozanski EA, Rush JE, et al. Association between outcome and organ system dysfunction in dogs with sepsis: 114 cases (2003–2007). J Am Vet Med Assoc 2010;236(1):83–7.
10. Kumar A, Parrillo JE. Myocardial depression in sepsis and septic shock. In: Abraham E, Singer M, editors. Mechanisms of sepsis-induced organ dysfunction and recovery. New York: Springer; 2007. p. 415–34.
11. Wiggers CJ. Myocardial depression in shock; a survey of cardiodynamic studies. Am Heart J 1947;33(5):633–50.
12. Waisbren BA. Bacteremia due to gram-negative bacilli other than the Salmonella; a clinical and therapeutic study. AMA Arch Intern Med 1951;88(4):467–88.
13. Lefer AM. Mechanisms of cardiodepression in endotoxin shock. Circ Shock Suppl 1979;1:1–8.
14. Parrillo JE, Burch C, Shelhamer JH, et al. A circulating myocardial depressant substance in humans with septic shock. Septic shock patients with a reduced ejection fraction have a circulating factor that depresses in vitro myocardial cell performance. J Clin Invest 1985;76(4):1539–53.
15. Price S, Anning PB, Mitchell JA, et al. Myocardial dysfunction in sepsis: mechanisms and therapeutic implications. Eur Heart J 1999;20(10):715–24.
16. Medzhitov R, Preston-Hurlburt P, Janeway CA Jr. A human homologue of the Drosophila Toll protein signals activation of adaptive immunity. Nature 1997; 388(6640):394–7.
17. Frantz S, Ertl G, Bauersachs J. Mechanisms of disease: toll-like receptors in cardiovascular disease. Nat Clin Pract Cardiovasc Med 2007;4(8):444–54.
18. Knapp S. Update on the role of Toll-like receptors during bacterial infections and sepsis. Wien Med Wochenschr 2010;160(5–6):107–11.
19. Leon CG, Tory R, Jia J, et al. Discovery and development of toll-like receptor 4 (TLR4) antagonists: a new paradigm for treating sepsis and other diseases. Pharm Res 2008;25(8):1751–61.

20. Tavener SA, Long EM, Robbins SM, et al. Immune cell Toll-like receptor 4 is required for cardiac myocyte impairment during endotoxemia. Circ Res 2004; 95(7):700–7.
21. Granton JT, Goddard CM, Allard MF, et al. Leukocytes and decreased left-ventricular contractility during endotoxemia in rabbits. Am J Respir Crit Care Med 1997;155(6):1977–83.
22. Tavener SA, Kubes P. Cellular and molecular mechanisms underlying LPS-associated myocyte impairment. Am J Physiol Heart Circ Physiol 2006;290(2): H800–6.
23. Binck BW, Tsen MF, Islas M, et al. Bone marrow-derived cells contribute to contractile dysfunction in endotoxic shock. Am J Physiol Heart Circ Physiol 2005;288(2):H577–83.
24. Knuefermann P, Sakata Y, Baker JS, et al. Toll-like receptor 2 mediates Staphylococcus aureus-induced myocardial dysfunction and cytokine production in the heart. Circulation 2004;110(24):3693–8.
25. Zou L, Feng Y, Chen YJ, et al. Toll-like receptor 2 plays a critical role in cardiac dysfunction during polymicrobial sepsis. Crit Care Med 2010;38(5):1335–42.
26. Knuefermann P, Schwederski M, Velten M, et al. Bacterial DNA induces myocardial inflammation and reduces cardiomyocyte contractility: role of toll-like receptor 9. Cardiovasc Res 2008;78(1):26–35.
27. Palsson-McDermott EM, O'Neill LA. Signal transduction by the lipopolysaccharide receptor, Toll-like receptor-4. Immunology 2004;113(2):153–62.
28. Shimazu R, Akashi S, Ogata H, et al. MD-2, a molecule that confers lipopolysaccharide responsiveness on Toll-like receptor 4. J Exp Med 1999;189(11):1777–82.
29. Visintin A, Mazzoni A, Spitzer JA, et al. Secreted MD-2 is a large polymeric protein that efficiently confers lipopolysaccharide sensitivity to Toll-like receptor 4. Proc Natl Acad Sci U S A 2001;98(21):12156–61.
30. Nozaki N, Shishido T, Takeishi Y, et al. Modulation of doxorubicin-induced cardiac dysfunction in toll-like receptor-2-knockout mice. Circulation 2004;110(18): 2869–74.
31. Riad A, Bien S, Gratz M, et al. Toll-like receptor-4 deficiency attenuates doxorubicin-induced cardiomyopathy in mice. Eur J Heart Fail 2008;10(3):233–43.
32. Barton GM, Medzhitov R. Toll-like receptor signaling pathways. Science 2003; 300(5625):1524–5.
33. Massey CV, Kohout TA, Gaa ST, et al. Molecular and cellular actions of platelet-activating factor in rat heart cells. J Clin Invest 1991;88(6):2106–16.
34. Yokoyama T, Vaca L, Rossen RD, et al. Cellular basis for the negative inotropic effects of tumor necrosis factor-alpha in the adult mammalian heart. J Clin Invest 1993;92(5):2303–12.
35. Heard SO, Toth IE, Perkins MW, et al. The role of protein kinase C in lipopolysaccharide-induced myocardial depression in guinea pigs. Shock 1994;1(6):419–24.
36. Oral H, Dorn GW, Mann DL. Sphingosine mediates the immediate negative inotropic effects of tumor necrosis factor-alpha in the adult mammalian cardiac myocyte. J Biol Chem 1997;272(8):4836–42.
37. Sugishita K, Kinugawa K, Shimizu T, et al. Cellular basis for the acute inhibitory effects of IL-6 and TNF- alpha on excitation-contraction coupling. J Mol Cell Cardiol 1999;31(8):1457–67.
38. Zhong J, Hwang TC, Adams HR, et al. Reduced L-type calcium current in ventricular myocytes from endotoxemic guinea pigs. Am J Physiol 1997;273(5 Pt 2): H2312–24.

39. Liu S, Schreur KD. G protein-mediated suppression of L-type Ca2+ current by interleukin-1 beta in cultured rat ventricular myocytes. Am J Physiol 1995;268 (2 Pt 1):C339–49.
40. Tavernier B, Garrigue D, Boulle C, et al. Myofilament calcium sensitivity is decreased in skinned cardiac fibres of endotoxin-treated rabbits. Cardiovasc Res 1998;38(2):472–9.
41. Tavernier B, Mebazaa A, Mateo P, et al. Phosphorylation-dependent alteration in myofilament Ca2+ sensitivity but normal mitochondrial function in septic heart. Am J Respir Crit Care Med 2001;163(2):362–7.
42. Ren J, Wu S. A burning issue: do sepsis and systemic inflammatory response syndrome (SIRS) directly contribute to cardiac dysfunction? Front Biosci 2006; 11:15–22.
43. Davani EY, Dorscheid DR, Lee CH, et al. Novel regulatory mechanism of cardio-myocyte contractility involving ICAM-1 and the cytoskeleton. Am J Physiol Heart Circ Physiol 2004;287(3):H1013–22.
44. Davani EY, Boyd JH, Dorscheid DR, et al. Cardiac ICAM-1 mediates leukocyte-dependent decreased ventricular contractility in endotoxemic mice. Cardiovasc Res 2006;72(1):134–42.
45. Ao L, Song Y, Fullerton DA, et al. The interaction between myocardial depressant factors in endotoxemic cardiac dysfunction: role of TNF-alpha in TLR4-mediated ICAM-1 expression. Cytokine 2007;38(3):124–9.
46. Pacher P, Beckman JS, Liaudet L. Nitric oxide and peroxynitrite in health and disease. Physiol Rev 2007;87(1):315–424.
47. dos Santos CC, Gattas DJ, Tsoporis JN, et al. Sepsis-induced myocardial depression is associated with transcriptional changes in energy metabolism and contractile related genes: a physiological and gene expression-based approach. Crit Care Med 2010;38(3):894–902.
48. Werdan K, Schmidt H, Ebelt H, et al. Impaired regulation of cardiac function in sepsis, SIRS, and MODS. Can J Physiol Pharmacol 2009;87(4):266–74.
49. Dunser MW, Hasibeder WR. Sympathetic overstimulation during critical illness: adverse effects of adrenergic stress. J Intensive Care Med 2009;24(5):293–316.
50. Zorn-Pauly K, Pelzmann B, Lang P, et al. Endotoxin impairs the human pace-maker current If. Shock 2007;28(6):655–61.
51. Rivers E, Nguyen B, Havstad S, et al. Early goal-directed therapy in the treatment of severe sepsis and septic shock. N Engl J Med 2001;345(19):1368–77.
52. Schmidt GA. Counterpoint: adherence to early goal-directed therapy: does it really matter? No. Both risks and benefits require further study. Chest 2010; 138(3):480–3.
53. Simmons JP, Wohl JS. Vasoactive catecholamines. In: Silverstein DC, Hopper K, editors. Small animal critical care medicine. St Louis (MO): Saunders Elsevier; 2009. p. 756–8.
54. Silverstein DC. Vasopressin. In: Silverstein DC, Hopper K, editors. Small animal critical care medicine. St Louis (MO): Saunders Elsevier; 2009. p. 759–62.
55. Annane D, Bellissant E, Bollaert PE, et al. Corticosteroids in the treatment of severe sepsis and septic shock in adults: a systematic review. JAMA 2009; 301(22):2362–75.
56. Wittebole X, Castanares-Zapatero D, Laterre PF. Toll-like receptor 4 modulation as a strategy to treat sepsis. Mediators Inflamm 2010;2010:568396.

The Kidney in Critically Ill Small Animals

Katharine F. Lunn, BVMS, MS, PhD, MRCVS

KEYWORDS

- Kidney • Azotemia • Uremia • Acute renal failure
- Acute kidney injury

This article discusses kidney disease in critically ill small animal patients. Critically ill patients may present to the clinician with kidney disease as the primary complaint, or kidney damage or dysfunction may arise as a complication or consequence of other illness. In the latter scenario, the clinician must carefully monitor parameters that assess renal function and be prepared to intervene to prevent irreversible injury.

NORMAL RENAL FUNCTION

The functions of the kidney are wide-ranging and critical for maintaining homeostasis. These functions include the regulation of electrolyte and acid-base balance, regulation of water balance, regulation of arterial blood pressure, excretion of metabolic wastes, excretion of hormones and exogenous compounds (eg, drugs), production of erythropoietin, synthesis of active vitamin D, and gluconeogenesis.[1]

The basic functional unit of the kidney is the nephron, which consists of the glomerulus, Bowman's capsule, and the renal tubule.[1] The glomerulus is interposed between an afferent and efferent arteriole within the renal cortex, and is the site of filtration of water and solutes from the blood. This filtrate passes into Bowman's space and then is significantly altered as it traverses the renal tubule. The functions of the different segments of the renal tubule are reflected in the functional and structural specializations of the epithelial cells that line the tubule.

Central to the function of the kidney is the unique blood supply to this organ. The kidneys receive approximately 20% of cardiac output,[2] all of which passes through the glomeruli. The blood enters the glomeruli through the afferent arterioles, 20% of the plasma passes into Bowman's space, and 80% of the plasma leaves through the efferent arterioles. Of the blood leaving the glomerulus, 90% or more passes through the peritubular capillaries in the renal cortex and into the renal venous system. The remaining 5% to 10% flows into the medulla through the vasa recta. These bundles of parallel vessels play an important role in solute and water exchange in

The author discloses no financial support relevant to this manuscript.
Department of Clinical Sciences, Colorado State University, 300 West Drake Road, Fort Collins, CO 80523-1620, USA
E-mail address: kathy.lunn@colostate.edu

the renal medullary interstitium. Although an in-depth review of renal vasculature, blood flow, glomerular filtration, and tubular function is beyond the scope of this article, an understanding of this area is important in understanding the role of the kidney in critical illness. The following facts are particularly noteworthy:

1. The vasculature of the renal cortex is highly unusual in that there are 2 arterioles (afferent and efferent) and 2 capillary beds (the glomerulus and the peritubular capillaries).
2. Glomerular filtration rate (GFR) reflects renal function.
3. The main factors affecting GFR are the permeability of the glomerular capillaries, the hydrostatic pressure in Bowman's capsule, the oncotic pressure of the blood, and the hydraulic pressure in the glomerular capillaries.
4. The pressure in the glomerular capillaries is determined by the pressure in 2 arterioles that are in series: the afferent and efferent arterioles. Changes in the resistance of each of these arterioles allow the kidney to regulate GFR independently of renal blood flow. For example, if renal arterial pressure falls, constriction of the efferent arteriole will increase the pressure in the glomerulus, and preserve GFR.
5. Constriction of the afferent or efferent arteriole has opposite effects on GFR, but both decrease renal blood flow. Changes in renal blood flow are important because they affect the metabolic functions and the integrity of the tubules. Changes in GFR affect excretion of water and solutes.
6. The kidney has a remarkable ability to maintain renal blood flow and glomerular filtration within a narrow range in the face of alterations in mean arterial blood pressure. This effectively isolates the kidney from normal fluctuations in systemic blood pressure and allows the kidney to continue its necessary homeostatic functions. This property is known as autoregulation and is effective over mean arterial blood pressures ranging from 70 to 170 mm Hg.
7. As noted earlier, the renal cortex receives about 90% of renal blood flow, with the medulla receiving about 10%, which means that the cortex is particularly vulnerable to blood-borne toxins.[2] In contrast, the medulla is more susceptible to ischemia.
8. Within the renal cortex, the most metabolically active nephron segments are most susceptible to ischemic damage, including the proximal tubule and the thick ascending limb of the loop of Henle.[2]
9. The processes that alter the ultrafiltrate in the nephron tend to concentrate nephrotoxins.

AZOTEMIA, UREMIA, AND RENAL FAILURE

Azotemia is defined as an increase in serum creatinine or blood urea nitrogen (BUN) concentrations, or both.[3] Thus it is defined by the results of laboratory tests. Uremia literally means the presence of urine constituents in the blood, but the term is generally used to refer to the clinical signs that develop as azotemia worsens.[3] These clinical signs commonly include decreased appetite, vomiting, lethargy, and weight loss. As uremia progresses, affected patients may develop uremic gastritis, oral ulcers, and platelet dysfunction. Less common signs of severe uremia may include uremic pneumonitis, osteodystrophy, and encephalopathy. Other consequences of worsening renal function include polyuria/polydipsia, dehydration, electrolyte derangements, acidosis, anemia, systemic hypertension, and renal secondary hyperparathyroidism.[3]

Azotemia, renal insults, renal disease, or renal failure are often classified as prerenal, renal, or postrenal;[4] many patients may have a combination of more than 1 type of azotemia or renal insult. The term prerenal implies normal renal morphology with a functional decrease in GFR, which may arise through decreased cardiac output, hypovolemia, hypotension, dehydration, decreased effective circulating volume, decreased plasma oncotic pressure, increased blood viscosity, or occlusion or constriction of the renal artery. When considering azotemia, the term prerenal also refers to an increase in BUN caused by increased protein intake or gastrointestinal bleeding. Renal azotemia or renal disease implies that the kidney itself is compromised and unable to perform its normal functions. Intrinsic renal disease can arise through a variety of different insults, many of which are discussed later. Postrenal azotemia implies that BUN and creatinine are increased because the urine does not exit the body through the normal route. This condition can arise through obstruction within the urinary tract, or rupture of the tract with subsequent leakage of urine into the abdomen.

Differentiation Between Prerenal, Renal, and Postrenal Azotemia

It is essential for the clinician to always consider prerenal, renal, and postrenal causes whenever a patient is newly diagnosed with azotemia, or whenever a previously stable azotemic patient experiences an unexpected increase in BUN or creatinine. This requirement is crucial because it may be possible to improve or fully reverse the prerenal or postrenal components of the azotemia. There is a continuum of damage between prerenal and renal azotemia, and between postrenal and renal azotemia. While it is diagnostically helpful, it is also vital, to consider the 3 components of azotemia, because failure to consider, and attempt to correct, prerenal and postrenal azotemia will eventually lead to intrinsic renal damage. For example, complete ureteral obstruction by a calcium oxalate nephrolith in a cat will initially reduce GFR because of increased hydrostatic pressure in Bowman's capsule. In time, the pressure in the renal pelvis will lead to hydronephrosis and permanent damage to the renal parenchyma.[5] This patient will therefore progress from postrenal disease to intrinsic renal disease. Similarly, a sustained decrease in renal artery pressure, if less than the limits of autoregulation, will result in renal ischemia, renal tubular cell damage, and eventually acute intrinsic renal failure. In this case, it may be argued that the distinction between prerenal and renal azotemia is artificial,[6] because prerenal factors, if not addressed, can progress to cause renal damage.

A prerenal component of azotemia should be assumed if the patient has a history of excessive fluid losses or decreased fluid intake. A prerenal component is also likely to be present if the patient has clinical findings consistent with hypotension, hypovolemia, shock, dehydration, or inadequate peripheral perfusion. The clinician must therefore rely on the history and physical examination findings to ensure that prerenal azotemia is considered; there are few specific laboratory tests that can confirm the presence of prerenal azotemia. In some cases, examination of the BUN/creatinine ratio can raise suspicion of a prerenal component to the azotemia. Creatinine is freely filtered at the glomerulus, and is not significantly secreted or reabsorbed. Thus, serum creatinine levels are largely dependent on GFR. In contrast, urea is both secreted and reabsorbed, as well as freely filtered, and it plays an essential role in urine concentrating ability. In simple terms, urea can be considered to follow water in the distal renal tubule. In a state of hypovolemia, hypotension, or dehydration, the kidney attempts to conserve water through the actions of antidiuretic hormone (ADH), and the same water-conserving mechanisms also promote reabsorption of urea. Thus, when GFR is decreased by prerenal factors, both creatinine and BUN increase, but BUN may increase to a proportionally greater extent as the kidney attempts to conserve water.

Interpretation of urine specific gravity is helpful when determining whether a patient has renal azotemia. It is most important for the clinician to consider whether urine specific gravity is appropriate for the patient, not whether it is normal. Kidneys respond appropriately to changes in body water balance by producing urine that allows excess water to be excreted, or by allowing water to be conserved in the face of dehydration. Water balance depends on 3 components: normal thirst, normal number and function of nephrons, and the action of ADH at the distal nephron. In renal disease, once approximately 66% of functional nephron mass is lost, renal concentrating ability is lost because the remaining nephrons must handle larger amounts of filtered solute, and this contributes to an osmotic diuresis. However, many other factors affect renal concentrating ability. Abnormal water intake leads to the production of a nonconcentrated urine; similarly, fluid therapy decreases urine specific gravity. Many drugs act to increase urine output. For example, diuretics are specifically used for this purpose. Other medications, such as glucocorticoids, may interfere with the action of ADH. Disease processes also interfere with renal concentrating ability without necessarily causing intrinsic renal damage.[7] Examples include typical hypoadrenocorticism (Addison's disease), hypercalcemia, diabetes mellitus, hyperadrenocorticism, and diabetes insipidus. In summary, if a patient is azotemic and the urine is concentrated (specific gravity >1.035 in a dog and >1.045 in a cat), renal azotemia is unlikely. If a patient is azotemic and the urine is not appropriately concentrated, that patient may have renal disease, but the clinician should consider other causes of failure to concentrate the urine: fluid therapy, medications, and concurrent diseases that cause polyuria. If the urine is hyposthenuric, renal failure is not ruled out because failing kidneys do retain diluting ability. However, renal tubular failure alone does not cause hyposthenuria, and the clinician must consider the presence of additional disease processes.

Addison's disease is a classic example of a single disease that can cause a significant azotemia together with failure to appropriately concentrate the urine. A patient in an addisonian crisis is often azotemic because of the presence of marked hypovolemia, hypotension, and dehydration. This patient has prerenal azotemia. The urine is not appropriately concentrated because marked sodium (Na) depletion in this patient decreases the hypertonicity of the renal medulla, which is essential for the creation of a concentrated urine. The example of the patient with Addison's disease illustrates another important feature of prerenal azotemia: it can be completely resolved with appropriate therapy. Thus, aggressive fluid therapy to restore volume in the patient with Addison's disease typically completely resolves the azotemia within 24 to 48 hours. By appropriately correcting the prerenal component of azotemia, the clinician has shown that this patient does not have renal azotemia.

Postrenal azotemia can be considered to be a urine flow problem: the urine is not exiting the body because of obstruction to urine flow, or because of diversion as a result of a rupture of the duct system. Obstruction or rupture can occur at any level of the urinary tract. These problems are best diagnosed with imaging. In the case of urinary tract rupture, an effusion will be present. The creatinine and potassium (K) content of the effusion should be measured and compared with serum levels.[8] If the creatinine or K levels in the fluid are more than twice those in the serum, the effusion likely contains urine. Because urinary tract obstruction can occur at any level, this cannot be ruled out in the patient that is able to urinate. The obstruction may be partial, or at the level of 1 ureter or renal pelvis. The combination of both abdominal radiographs and abdominal ultrasound gives the best diagnostic accuracy for detection of urinary tract obstruction.[9] The obstruction of 1 kidney only leads to azotemia if the contralateral kidney is subnormal. The most common example of this scenario is ureteral obstruction in cats.[4] For the development of azotemia, approximately 75% of functional nephron mass must be lost. Thus ureteral obstruction does not cause azotemia if the remaining kidney is normal (because only 50% of renal mass has been lost). However, if ureteral obstruction occurs in a cat with preexisting renal disease, the remaining kidney may not be able to provide more than 25% of renal function, and azotemia will result. This patient has both renal and postrenal azotemia.

Many acutely azotemic patients have more then 1 type of azotemia. For example, the cat with ureterolithiasis described earlier may have preexisting chronic kidney disease causing renal azotemia, an obstructing ureterolith causing postrenal azotemia, and fluid deficits caused by anorexia and vomiting causing prerenal azotemia. It is the clinician's responsibility to consider all forms of azotemia and their appropriate therapies. In **Table 1**, clinical questions are used to frame the approach to the azotemic patient, ensuring that the clinician considers the different potential causes of azotemia, as well as the tools used to detect them.

Table 1
Clinical questions that frame the approach to the azotemic patient

Clinical Question	Important Findings	Recommended Therapy
Is the azotemia prerenal?	History Physical examination BUN/creatinine ratio	Fluid support Oncotic support Blood pressure support

Is the azotemia postrenal?	Abdominal radiographs
	Abdominal ultrasonography
	Abdominocentesis and fluid
	  analysis
		Surgical or medical therapy,
		  depending on cause

Is the azotemia renal?	History
	Response to therapy for
	  prerenal and postrenal
	  causes
	Urine specific gravity
		Address prerenal and
		  postrenal causes

Is renal azotemia acute
  or chronic or both?
	History
	Physical examination
	Packed cell volume
	Renal imaging
		Assume acute component
		  in the sick patient
		Provide therapy for acute
		  renal failure (see text)

If acute renal azotemia,
  is the cause a drug
  or toxin?
	History
	Specific testing where
	  applicable
		Remove drug or toxin
		Specific antidotes when
		  available

If acute renal azotemia,
  is the cause an infection?
	Urine culture
	Specific disease testing
		Antibiotics if pyelonephritis
		  suspected
		Antibiotics in a dog if
		  leptospirosisis not ruled
		  out or another specific
		  cause is not identified

What are the consequences
  of renal failure in this
  patient?
	Volume status
	Blood pressure
	Perfusion parameters
	Body weight
	Appetite
	Urine output
	Serum chemistry profile
	Blood gas/lactate
	Complete blood count
	Urinalysis
		Fluid therapy
		Pressor support
		Antihypertensive
		  medications
		Address electrolyte
		  abnormalities
		Address acid-base status
		Provide nutritional support

KIDNEY DISEASE

Kidney disease may be defined as structural or functional abnormalities in 1 or both kidneys.[3] Thus, a clinically insignificant renal cyst and catastrophic acute renal failure (ARF) caused by ethylene glycol intoxication are both examples of kidney disease. Disease of 1 or both kidneys may be detected by laboratory testing (including blood and urine tests), histopathologic examination of tissue, or imaging studies such as radiographs or ultrasonography. The severity of renal disease and the implications for therapy and prognosis can vary between patients. Many of the terms used to describe kidney disease are confusing or poorly defined. One example is the term renal insufficiency. This may be interpreted to mean loss of renal concentrating ability in the absence of azotemia; it may be used to signify mild azotemia, or it may imply loss of renal reserve or an inability to compensate for further loss of renal function.

Poorly defined terms have led to attempts to standardize the language and terminology of kidney disease. The use of consistent definitions should allow clearer communication and recording of clinical findings, and also more meaningful comparisons between research studies.

Chronic Kidney Disease: Definition and Staging

The international renal interest society (IRIS; www.iris-kidney.com) has proposed that the term chronic kidney disease (CKD) be used in preference to chronic renal failure. In this context, chronic implies the presence of kidney damage for at least 3 months.[3] This time course is typically inferred from historical findings or from the results of repeated laboratory tests that show persistent azotemia or abnormalities on urinalysis. Historical findings in chronic renal failure may include polyuria/polydipsia, weight loss, decreased appetite, and lethargy. The chronicity of the disease process may be supported by the presence of a nonregenerative anemia, or by the appearance of the kidneys or radiographs or ultrasound examination.

CKD may be defined as:

1. Kidney damage present for at least 3 months, with or without a decrease in GFR, or
2. A reduction in GFR by more than 50% below normal, present for at least 3 months.[3]

CKD is then staged from the fasting creatinine value assessed on at least 2 occasions in the stable patient, which implies that a CKD stage is not usually assigned at the initial time diagnosis of kidney disease, and, more importantly, a CKD stage should not be applied to a patient that is not clinically stable. **Table 2** summarizes the IRIS stages of CKD in dogs and cats. This system allows for primary staging based on serum creatinine values. Additional substages are then assigned depending on the level of proteinuria present and the patient's blood pressure.

Table 2
IRIS stages of CKD in dogs and cats

Stage	Serum Creatinine Value (mg/dL)		Azotemia
	Dogs	Cats	
1	<1.4	<1.6	Nonazotemic
2	1.4–2.0	1.6–2.8	Mild azotemia
3	2.1–5.0	2.9–5.0	Moderate azotemia
4	≥5.0	≥5.0	Severe azotemia

ARF and Acute Kidney Injury

Many definitions of ARF can be found in the veterinary literature, such as:

- The sudden inability of the kidneys to regulate water and solute balance[10]
- Rapid deterioration of renal function resulting in the accumulation of nitrogenous wastes such as urea and creatinine[10]
- An abrupt and prolonged decline in glomerular filtration resulting in the accumulation of nitrogenous wastes.[11]

The elements that these definitions have in common are that renal failure occurs in a short time period, and that there is a consequent loss of renal function. Some of these definitions also state, or imply, that BUN and/or creatinine are increased beyond the reference range in ARF. What is less clear from these definitions is the nature of the other renal functions that are affected, the methods by which these functions are assessed, and the amount of deviation from normal that is considered significant. The terms sudden, rapid, abrupt, and prolonged are also not clearly defined.

In human medicine, the term acute kidney injury (AKI) is gradually replacing ARF,[12–14] and classification schemes are used to define the severity and outcome of AKI in people. One example of such a scheme is a multilevel classification system[15–17] that defines 3 levels of severity of AKI: risk (R), injury (I), and failure (F) based on objective measurement of serum creatinine and/or GFR, and urine output. The criteria also allow for 2 levels of outcome of AKI: loss of function (L) and end-stage renal disease (E). This system is known as the RIFLE classification scheme, and it is summarized in **Table 3**. By replacing the term ARF with AKI, proponents of the RIFLE classification system have suggested that the entire spectrum of acute changes in renal function is included in the definition. The use of the classification system provides a more uniform definition of AKI, and this should facilitate a more uniform approach to diagnosis, therapy, and prognosis. It should also assist in the design and interpretation of studies of AKI in clinical patients.[13]

Classification schemes for AKI have not yet been broadly adopted in veterinary medicine, although a scoring system has been proposed to facilitate prediction of the outcome of hemodialysis in dogs with AKI.[18] Examination of **Table 3** reveals at least 2 significant reasons why this scheme would be difficult to apply to veterinary

Table 3
RIFLE classification scheme for AKI in human patients

	GFR and Creatinine	Urine Output
Severity Category		
R (risk)	↑ Creatinine×1.5, or GFR ↓ >25%	UO <0.5 mL/kg/h ×6 h
I (injury)	↑ Creatinine×2, or GFR ↓ >50%	UO <0.5 mL/kg/h ×12 h
F (failure)	↑ Creatinine×3, or GFR ↓ 75%, or creatinine >4 mg/dL, or acute ↑ creatinine ≥0.5 mg/dL	UO <0.3 mL/kg/h ×24 h, or anuria×12 h
Outcome Category		
L (loss)	Persistent ARF = complete loss of kidney function >4 wk	
E (end-stage kidney disease)	End-stage kidney disease >3 mo	

Abbreviations: GFR, glomerular filtration rate; UO, urine output.
Data from Bellomo R, Ronco C, Kellum JA, et al. Acute renal failure - definition, outcome measures, animal models, fluid therapy and information technology needs: the Second International Consensus Conference of the Acute Dialysis Quality Initiative (ADQI) Group. Crit Care 2004;8(4):R206.

patients: baseline creatinine values are rarely known, and urine output is not routinely measured. The term AKI is also not consistently applied in veterinary patients. Most clinicians are more comfortable with the term ARF. Because strict definitions have yet to be agreed on in veterinary medicine, AKI and ARF are used interchangeably in this article.

PATHOPHYSIOLOGY OF ARF

ARF is frequently described in 4 stages: initiation, extension, maintenance, and recovery.[4] It is not always possible to distinguish clinically between these phases. The initiation phase begins with the renal insult and continues until there is a detectable change in renal function. Intervention during this phase may prevent progression. In the extension phase, the initial renal insult is amplified by ongoing renal inflammation and hypoxia. In the maintenance phase, there is little normal tubular function, GFR is decreased, and a critical amount of irreversible damage has occurred. In the recovery phase, the renal tissue regenerates and repairs. In patients that survive ARF, this phase is often identified by the development of a significant polyuria. During this phase it is important to avoid any further renal insults.

Both ischemic renal damage and nephrotoxins lead to pathologic changes in the kidney known as acute tubular necrosis.[19] Although still widely used, this term is inaccurate, because necrosis of tubular cells is not a consistent finding.[20] A full description of the cellular and molecular events underlying acute tubular necrosis is beyond the scope of this article. However, an appreciation for the changes that occur can help the clinician understand the rationale behind the common therapeutic interventions that are indicated in the prevention and management of ARF.

When the pressure in the renal artery decreases to below the autoregulatory range, constriction of the afferent arteriole reduces glomerular filtration pressure and GFR (leading to prerenal azotemia). Blood flow also decreases in the postglomerular capillaries and, as this worsens, ischemia leads to renal tubular damage. Oxygen depletion in the renal tubular cells leads to cytoskeletal disruption, with resultant sloughing of intact cells and cellular debris into the tubular lumen. Cytoskeletal disruption also causes mislocation of the Na/K-ATPase from the basolateral to the apical cell membrane, thus disrupting sodium transport. The ensuing high Na concentration in the tubule causes Tam-Horsfall protein polymerization. The net result of these changes is that the renal tubules become occluded by cellular and protein casts and debris. This occlusion increases intratubular hydrostatic pressure and reduces GFR. Glomerular filtrate also leaks across the denuded tubular walls into the capillaries, further reducing the effective GFR and contributing to azotemia. Other factors involved in the pathophysiology of ARF include intrarenal vasoconstriction, renal medullary hypoxia, and neutrophil chemotaxis with associated release of damaging enzymes and inflammatory mediators.[20]

CAUSES OF ARF

In human medicine, ischemia and nephrotoxin exposure are the most common causes of ARF.[21] Hospital-acquired ARF is a significant problem in human medicine, particularly in the intensive care unit (ICU), and it is frequently multifactorial.[14] Considering both hospital-acquired and community-acquired causes of ARF in humans, approximately 50% of cases are caused by ischemia, 35% are caused by toxins, 10% are attributed to interstitial nephritis, and 5% to acute glomerulonephritis.[21]

In contrast with the wealth of data regarding causes of ARF in human patients, there are few studies that document the relative frequency of the causes of ARF in dogs and cats. **Table 4** summarizes the causes of ARF in dogs and cats. In a retrospective study of ARF in 99 dogs presented to a large referral hospital, 33 patients were diagnosed with an isolated ischemic event, the most common of which was pancreatitis (9 cases), 21 dogs were exposed to a single nephrotoxicant (including 12 cases of ethylene glycol toxicosis), 4 dogs had an infectious cause (leptospirosis or pyelonephritis), and 18 dogs had multiple disorders. Of the dogs with multiple disorders, 10 dogs had disseminated intravascular coagulation (DIC) in conjunction with another disease and 5 dogs had pancreatitis in conjunction with another disease. In 22 of the dogs in this case series, no cause for the ARF could be identified.[11]

A recently published case series documented the causes of naturally-acquired ARF in 32 cats.[22] Nephrotoxicosis was the most common cause, accounting for 18 cases (56%). Nine of these were caused by lily ingestion. Four cats had experienced ischemic events, including 2 patients that underwent general anesthesia. The remaining 10 cats had suspected pyelonephritis or ARF of unknown cause.

Community-acquired ARF

In human medicine, prerenal causes account for about 70% of cases of community-acquired ARF.[21] Common causes include excessive fluid losses caused by gastrointestinal disease, inadequate fluid intake, heart failure, and use of diuretics.

In the canine case series summarized earlier,[11] it is not clear how many dogs had community-acquired ARF and how many had hospital-acquired ARF. It is possible that some of the ischemic events occurred in hospitalized patients before referral. Nonetheless, this case series suggests that most cases of community-acquired ARF in dogs likely result from ischemia or nephrotoxicant exposure, or are of unknown cause. In contrast, the feline case series indicates that nephrotoxicants are the most common cause of ARF in cats, although this is based on a small number of cases.[22]

Hospital-acquired ARF

Hospital-acquired ARF in humans is often the result of multiple renal insults, with frequent contributions from hypovolemia, sepsis, and nephrotoxic medications.[14] A multicenter study of almost 30,000 human patients in ICUs revealed that the 5 most common causes of ARF were sepsis, major surgery, low cardiac output, hypovolemia, and medications.[23] There is only 1 published study documenting the causes of hospital-acquired ARF in dogs, and there are no studies involving cats. In the study on dogs, a retrospective case series identified hospital-acquired ARF in 29 dogs.[24] The most common inciting causes identified were nephrotoxicosis in 21 dogs (72%), advanced age ($\geq$7 years) in 20 dogs (69%), chronic heart disease (12 dogs; 41%) and preexisting renal disease (9 dogs; 31%). The most common nephrotoxicants were aminoglycoside antibiotics, cardiac medications, and cisplatin. The overall mortality in this case series was high at 62%. Older dogs appeared to be at greater risk of developing hospital-acquired ARF, and were more likely to subsequently die. Although small, this case series is important because it highlights that some of the inciting causes of hospital-acquired ARF are within the control of the veterinarian. Aging is inevitable, but medications can be chosen and used with care.

A recent multicenter retrospective case series examined organ dysfunction in dogs with sepsis caused by gastrointestinal tract lesions.[25] The study revealed that multiple organ dysfunction syndrome can be identified in these patients, and that organ dysfunction increased the odds of death. Renal dysfunction, as well as respiratory, cardiovascular, or coagulation disorders, was found to independently increase the odds of death. Thus prevention of hospital-acquired ARF is likely to improve patient survival.

Table 4
Selected causes of ARF in small animals

Prerenal and Postrenal Causes	Endogenous Nephrotoxins	Exogenous Nephrotoxins: Drugs and Medical Interventions	Exogenous Nephrotoxins: Environmental	Infectious, Inflammatory, Neoplastic, and Miscellaneous Causes
Hypovolemia	Myoglobin	Aminoglycosides	Ethylene glycol	Leptospirosis (D)
Hypotension	Hemoglobin	Cephalosporins	Lilies (C)	Pyelonephritis
Sepsis	Hypercalcemia	Tetracyclines	Grapes, raisins, currants (D)	Lyme disease (D)
MODS		Other antibiotics	Melamine/cyanuric acid	Rocky Mountain spotted fever (D)
Decreased cardiac output		Amphotericin B	Snake venom	Ehrlichiosis (D)
Renal artery disease		Thiacetarsemide	Heavy metals	Other systemic bacterial infections
Other causes of ischemia		Cisplatin	Chlorinated hydrocarbons	Glomerulonephritis
Urethral obstruction		Doxorubicin		Amyloidosis
Ureteral obstruction		Vincristine		Systemic lupus erythematosus
		Other cytotoxic drugs		Vasculitis
		Cyclosporine		Transplant rejection
		NSAIDs		Lymphosarcoma
		Diuretics		Other neoplasia
		ACE inhibitors		Trauma
		Methylene blue		
		Radiocontrast agents		

Abbreviations: ACE, angiotensin-converting enzyme; C, cats; D, dogs; MODS, multiple organ dysfunction syndrome; NSAID, nonsteroidal antiinflammatory drug.

NORMOTENSIVE ISCHEMIC ARF

As noted earlier, ischemia is one of the most common causes of ARF in humans, and, in many of these patients, there is an obvious inciting cause, such as sepsis, surgery, heart disease, or hypovolemia. However, in some cases, systemic hypotension is not detected, and ischemia seems to result from increased renal susceptibility to modest reductions in perfusion pressure. This condition is called normotensive ischemic ARF and is associated with conditions in which autoregulation is impaired.[20] The healthy kidney is able to maintain GFR in the face of systemic hypotension by decreasing afferent arteriolar resistance. This mechanism may be ineffective in patients with atherosclerosis, hypertension, or chronic renal failure, because of structural narrowing of the arterioles. Failure to decrease afferent arteriolar resistance is also the mechanism by which nonsteroidal antiinflammatory drugs (NSAIDs) can lead to ARF, because these drugs inhibit the synthesis of renal vasodilatory prostaglandins. Other causes of increased afferent arteriolar resistance include sepsis, hypercalcemia, and radiocontrast agents. When renal perfusion pressure decreases, GFR is also maintained by constriction of the efferent arteriole. In patients receiving angiotensin-converting enzyme (ACE) inhibitors or angiotensin receptor blockers, this protective mechanism is diminished, and moderate decreases in renal perfusion may lead to ARF. Hypertension, chronic renal failure, and sepsis may all occur in critically ill small animals, and these patients may also be receiving NSAIDs or ACE inhibitors.[2] Thus, it is reasonable to assume that normotensive ischemic ARF may also occur in dogs and cats.

PREVENTION OF HOSPITAL-ACQUIRED ARF

Several steps are necessary to minimize the risk of ARF in hospitalized patients. These steps can be summarized as follows:

Awareness of Risk Factors for ARF

Risk factors for ARF in small animal patients are presented in **Table 5**. Some of these factors are beyond the control of the clinician (examples include preexisting renal disease and age), which emphasizes how important it is to be aware of the risk factors that are within the control of the clinician, so that they may be minimized or avoided. In addition, risk factors are likely to be additive. For example, the use of an aminoglycoside antibiotic in a normovolemic young animal is likely to be associated with a lower risk of nephrotoxicity than the use of that same drug in an elderly patient that is volume-depleted because of chronic vomiting. In this example, an alternate antibiotic should be used; and, if this is not possible, the aminoglycoside should be used in conjunction with therapeutic drug monitoring and should not be administered until all volume and electrolyte deficits have been addressed.

Management of Risk Factors for ARF

Crystalloid and colloid fluid therapy should be used in critically ill patients to prevent or treat volume and hydration deficits and maintain renal perfusion. Patients undergoing general anesthesia should receive fluid therapy. Intravenous fluids can be used to reduce the risk associated with other necessary procedures. For example, use of crystalloid fluid therapy may reduce the risk of ARF caused by contrast-induced nephropathy.[26] Fluids can also be used to correct electrolyte and acid-base disorders. Blood pressure monitoring is essential in critically ill patients, and pressors should be used if necessary. Hypertension should also be corrected because this is directly damaging to the kidneys, as well as other end-organs such as the heart and central

Table 5 Potential risk factors for ARF		
Concurrent Conditions	**Correctable Abnormalities**	**Potentially Avoidable Interventions**
Preexisting renal disease	Dehydration	Radiocontrast agents
Advancing age	Hypotension	Anesthesia
Cardiac disease	Hypertension	Surgery
Fever	Decreased cardiac	Nephrotoxic drugs:
Sepsis	output	(A) Intrinsically nephrotoxic (eg,
Liver disease	Decreased colloid	aminoglycosides, cisplatin)
Pancreatitis	oncotic pressure	(B) Increased risk of ARF in
Neoplasia	Hyponatremia	combination with other
Trauma	Hypokalemia	factors (eg, NSAIDs, ACE inhibitors)
Burns	Hypercalcemia	(C) Inappropriate drug combinations
Vasculitis	Hypocalcemia	(eg, furosemide and gentamicin)
MODS	Hypomagnesemia	
Diabetes mellitus	Acidosis	
Hypoalbuminemia		
Multiple myeloma		
Hemoglobinuria		
Myoglobinuria		

Abbreviation: MODS, multiple organ dysfunction syndrome.

nervous system. Nephrotoxic medications should be avoided if possible, and particular attention should be paid to potentially harmful drug combinations. For example, an elderly patient that is receiving a combination of an NSAID with an ACE inhibitor is at greater risk of developing ARF as a result of severe hydration or volume deficits. Antibiotic choices should be based on the results of bacterial culture and sensitivity testing. If the results of those are not available, the clinician should consider the site of infection and the organisms that are suspected before antibiotic selection. In critically ill patients, particularly those with sepsis, broad-spectrum antibiotic therapy is often used. If aminoglycoside therapy is necessary, it is recommended that a once-daily dosing schedule is followed,[27] and that urine is monitored for early markers of renal damage (see later discussion). Monitoring of BUN and creatinine is not sensitive enough for this purpose.

Early Detection of ARF

In human medicine, serum creatinine levels are compared with baseline values, and urine output is measured to classify AKI, particularly when this develops in the ICU.[16] The RIFLE system uses these elements for classification (see **Table 3**). Veterinary patients may already be critically ill when initially hospitalized, and a true baseline creatinine value is therefore not available. However, daily monitoring of creatinine values in hospitalized patients may reveal trends that suggest declining renal function. Serum creatinine is a readily available test and it continues to be the primary tool used for assessment of renal function. Despite this, it is important to recognize that a single creatinine value can be an insensitive tool. A doubling of serum creatinine correlates with a loss of approximately 50% of GFR, or functional nephron mass.[1] Thus, with constant production, an increase in serum creatinine from 0.6 to 1.2 mg/dL represents a 50% decrease in GFR, although both values are within the reference range.

Measurement of urine output is sensitive to renal hemodynamics, and changes in urine output may precede changes in serum creatinine values. In human medicine, low urine output has a high positive predictive value for the development of ARF. However, good urine output does not rule out renal dysfunction, thus the negative predictive value is low.[16] Quantitation of urine output in small animal patients is most likely to occur in patients with a diagnosis of ARF, and in patients that are non-ambulatory and have a urinary catheter placed for ease of management. Consideration should be given to the monitoring of urine output in other critically ill patients that may be at risk for development of ARF.

Results of urinalysis and urine sediment examination can provide evidence of renal disease before significant changes in serum creatinine or urine output are observed. Examples include the presence of casts, pyuria, or bacteruria, and the presence of glycosuria in the absence of hyperglycemia.[28] For example, casts in the urine may signal aminoglycoside nephrotoxicity before there are changes in the serum creatinine.[29]

In addition to the standard urinalysis, measurement of urine electrolytes can provide further information about renal function. For example, fractional excretion of Na can be used to help distinguish between prerenal azotemia and intrinsic ARF in azotemic patients, although the distinction may not always be definitive in clinical patients.[30] Urinary Na and chloride levels may also be useful for detecting significant renal damage after suspected NSAID toxicity, and for monitoring for the development of aminoglycoside toxicity,[30] and in both of these situations, a value should be obtained on admission to the hospital or before administration of the potential nephrotoxin. Serial measurements may then detect renal damage.

Detection and measurement of enzymuria (enzymes in the urine) has also been used for early detection of renal injury.[31] These are typically molecules that are too large to be filtered at the glomerulus, and therefore their appearance in the urine may indicate leakage from damaged tubular cells. For example, γ-glutamyl transferase (GGT) and N-acetyl-β-D-glucosaminidase (NAG) both originate in proximal tubule cells, and measurement of their levels, sometimes expressed as a urine enzyme/creatinine ratio, has been used as a marker for aminoglycoside-induced renal damage.[29,32–34] These measurements are most useful when a baseline value is obtained before the use of aminoglyosides.[28,31] Other urinary markers that are being increasingly studied in dogs include C-reactive protein (CRP), immunoglobulin G (IgG), thromboxane B_2 (TXB$_2$), and retinol binding protein (RBP).[35,36] Both CRP and IgG are markers for glomerular damage, whereas RBP is a marker for proximal tubular damage, and TXB$_2$ levels may reflect intrarenal hemodynamics. Some of these markers have been used in experimental models of canine ARF,[37] but there is little information available regarding their clinical use in critically ill veterinary patients at risk for development of AKI.

MANAGEMENT OF ARF

When ARF is suspected or diagnosed, the following stepwise approach is suggested:

1. Obtain a detailed history.
   Determine whether the patient has been exposed to any potential nephrotoxicants, or has recently experienced anesthesia, surgery, or any other illness. Document all current and recently administered medications, including supplements and nutraceuticals.
2. Obtain baseline physical examination data.
   Assess volume, hydration, and perfusion parameters. Record temperature, pulse/heart rate, respiratory rate, arterial blood pressure, and body weight.

3. Obtain venous access.

A jugular catheter or peripherally inserted central catheter (PICC) is recommended, which allows measurement of central venous pressure (CVP), and a multiple lumen catheter facilitates repeated blood sampling for monitoring purposes. Record initial CVP, packed cell volume (PCV), and total solids (TS). Note: if the patient is likely to be referred for renal replacement therapy, the jugular veins should be preserved for that purpose.

4. Obtain baseline laboratory data.

Complete blood count, serum biochemistry profile, venous blood gas, and complete urinalysis should be performed. Urine should be saved for culture.

5. Correct fluid and volume deficits.

Calculate volume required for rehydration using body weight (in kilograms) times estimated dehydration (%), which gives fluid deficit in liters. The deficit should be corrected in 4 to 24 hours, depending on the patient's clinical status and ability to handle a fluid load. A buffered balanced electrolyte solution should be used initially, such as lactated Ringer's solution or Normosol. Consider colloidal support, if indicated.

6. Place a urinary catheter.

A urinary catheter with a closed collection system facilitates measurement of urine output. A urinary catheter is also important if leptospirosis is suspected, because it limits environmental exposure to potentially infectious urine. If placement of a urinary catheter is not possible, small dogs can be encouraged to urinate on absorbent pads that can be weighed to assess urine output, and cats can be provided with litter boxes containing nonabsorbent litter.

7. Treat the treatable and test for the testable.

Stop any potentially nephrotoxic medications. Submit urine for aerobic culture. Perform testing for leptospirosis in all dogs with ARF. Test for ethylene glycol, if indicated.

Obtain abdominal radiographs and ultrasound to rule out postrenal azotemia, once the patient is stable. Administer antibiotics if leptospirosis is not ruled out in a dog and if pyelonephritis is suspected in a dog or cat. Consider antidotes for ethylene glycol ingestion as soon as possible, if there is a possibility of exposure.

8. Determine urine output.

Once the fluid deficit has been corrected, urine output (UOP) should be quantified and expressed as milliliters per kilogram body weight per hour. Determine whether patient is polyuric (UOP>2 mL/kg/h), oliguric (UOP<1 mL/kg/h), or anuric (UOP = 0 mL/kg/h).

9. Correct anuria or oliguria.

If the patient is not overhydrated, an additional fluid load equal to 2% to 5% of body weight may be administered over 4 to 6 hours. If there is no increase in UOP, several other interventions should be considered, alone or in combination:

A. Administer mannitol as a bolus, followed by constant rate infusion (CRI). This step is contraindicated in patients that are volume overloaded.[38]

B. Administer furosemide as a bolus, followed by CRI. This step is often used in combination with dopamine.[38]

C. Administer dopamine by CRI, with blood pressure and electrocardiogram (ECG) monitoring.[38]

D. Consider diltiazem in dogs, given by CRI.[39]
E. Consider fenoldopam in cats, given by CRI.[40]
Note that the use of dopamine and furosemide, alone or in combination, has little support in the human literature.[41–43] There are few studies in the veterinary literature that address the value of these interventions in veterinary patients with anuric or oliguric renal failure. It is clear that conversion to a polyuric state allows ongoing fluid support and management of the patient with ARF, whereas failure to resolve anuria or oliguria necessitates the provision of continuous renal replacement therapy, peritoneal dialysis, or hemodialysis.

10. Provide ongoing fluid therapy.
For the polyuric patient, the fluid recipe should be calculated using the ins-and-outs method, and thus measurement of urine output is necessary. Urine output should be measured over a period of 2 to 6 hours, and the hourly output calculated. This hourly rate is added to insensible losses to give the total hourly rate of crystalloid fluids. Insensible losses are usually assumed to be 20 mL/kg/24 h. Additional losses such as vomiting or diarrhea should be measured or estimated, and added to the patient's fluid needs. The fluid requirement should be recalculated at least 4 times daily, and the accurate measurement of urine output is essential in the polyuric patient because the volume of urine produced can be unpredictable and high. The use of shortcuts such as twice maintenance or 3-times maintenance is discouraged. Failure to account for polyuria in these patients rapidly leads to a worsening fluid deficit with associated worsening of renal perfusion. The patient is driving the urine output, and the clinician must respond to this with administration of appropriate fluid volumes.

11. Monitor the patient:
A. Hydration status and body weight (at least twice daily)
B. CVP
C. Systemic blood pressure and perfusion parameters
D. Urine output
E. PCV/TS
F. Electrolytes
G. Acid-base parameters
H. Creatinine, BUN, and phosphorus.

12. Provide adequate nutrition.
Manage nausea and vomiting and address possible uremic gastritis. Use enteral nutrition whenever possible, using feeding tubes if necessary. If enteral nutrition is not tolerated, parenteral nutrition should be provided. Volumes administered enterally or parenterally should be accounted for in the fluid therapy recipe.

13. Address the consequences of renal failure.
Use phosphate binders for hyperphosphatemia to mitigate development of renal secondary hyperparathyroidism. Treat hypertension and address anemia.

14. Renal replacement therapy.
This should be considered for patients that remain anuric or oliguric, for patients with fluid overload or refractory electrolyte/acid-base abnormalities, and for patients with severe uremia that is not responsive to medical management. Options for renal replacement therapy include continuous renal replacement therapy, intermittent hemodialysis, and peritoneal dialysis.[18,44–47] These

options are available in few locations, and therefore clinicians should familiarize themselves with the options that are available in their practice area, and be prepared to discuss these interventions with clients at an early stage.

SUMMARY

Many risk factors for AKI are likely to be present in critically ill patients. Factors to consider include age, preexisting disease, concurrent medical therapy, electrolyte and fluid imbalances, and exposure to potential nephrotoxicants. Many risk factors are correctable or manageable, and these should be addressed whenever possible. In human patients in the ICU, the 5 most common causes of ARF are sepsis, major surgery, low cardiac output, hypovolemia, and medications. It is reasonable to assume that these are also important causes in veterinary medicine. Measurement of serum creatinine is an insensitive tool for the detection of AKI, and therefore clinicians should consider assessment of other parameters such as urine output, urinalysis, and urine chemistry results.

REFERENCES

1. Eaton DC, Pooler JP. Vander's renal physiology. 7th edition. New York: McGraw-Hill; 2009.
2. Grauer GF. Prevention of acute renal failure. Vet Clin North Am Small Anim Pract 1996;26(6):1447–59.
3. Polzin DJ. Chronic kidney disease. In: Ettinger SJ, Feldman EC, editors, Textbook of veterinary internal medicine, vol. 2. St Louis (MO): Saunders Elsevier; 2010. p. 1990–2021.
4. Langston C. Acute uremia. In: Ettinger SJ, Feldman EC, editors. 7th edition, Textbook of veterinary internal medicine, vol. 2. St Louis (MO): Saunders Elsevier; 2010. p. 1969–85.
5. Hardie EM, Kyles AE. Management of ureteral obstruction. Vet Clin North Am Small Anim Pract 2004;34(4):989–1010.
6. Bellomo R, Bagshaw S, Langenberg C, et al. Pre-renal azotemia: a flawed paradigm in critically ill septic patients? Contrib Nephrol 2007;156:1–9.
7. Cohen M, Post GS. Water transport in the kidney and nephrogenic diabetes insipidus. J Vet Intern Med 2002;16(5):510–7.
8. Schmeidt C, Tobias KM, Otto CM. Evaluation of abdominal fluid: peripheral blood creatinine and potassium ratios for diagnosis of uroperitoneum in dogs. J Vet Emerg Crit Care 2001;11:275–80.
9. Kyles AE, Hardie EM, Wooden BG, et al. Clinical, clinicopathologic, radiographic, and ultrasonographic abnormalities in cats with ureteral calculi: 163 cases (1984–2002). J Am Vet Med Assoc 2005;226(6):932–6.
10. Labato MA. Strategies for management of acute renal failure. Vet Clin North Am Small Anim Pract 2001;31(6):1265–87, vii.
11. Vaden SL, Levine J, Breitschwerdt EB. A retrospective case-control of acute renal failure in 99 dogs. J Vet Intern Med 1997;11(2):58–64.
12. Mehta RL, Kellum JA, Shah SV, et al. Acute kidney injury network: report of an initiative to improve outcomes in acute kidney injury. Crit Care 2007;11(2):R31.
13. Kellum JA. Acute kidney injury. Crit Care Med 2008;36(Suppl):S141–5.
14. Dennen P, Douglas IS, Anderson R. Acute kidney injury in the intensive care unit: an update and primer for the intensivist. Crit Care Med 2010;38(1):261–75.
15. Bellomo R, Ronco C, Kellum JA, et al. Acute renal failure - definition, outcome measures, animal models, fluid therapy and information technology needs: the

Second International Consensus Conference of the Acute Dialysis Quality Initiative (ADQI) Group. Crit Care 2004;8(4):R204–12.

16. Venkataraman R, Kellum JA. Defining acute renal failure: the RIFLE criteria. J Intensive Care Med 2007;22(4):187–93.

17. Kellum JA. Defining and classifying AKI: one set of criteria. Nephrol Dial Transplant 2008;23(5):1471–2.

18. Segev G, Kass PH, Francey T, et al. A novel clinical scoring system for outcome prediction in dogs with acute kidney injury managed by dialysis. J Vet Intern Med 2008;22:301–8.

19. Lameire NL. The pathophysiology of acute renal failure. Crit Care Clin 2005;21: 197–210.

20. Abuelo JG. Normotensive ischemic acute renal failure. N Engl J Med 2007; 357(8):797–805.

21. Thadhani R, Pascual M, Bonventre JV. Acute renal failure. N Engl J Med 1996; 334(22):1448–60.

22. Worwag S, Langston CE. Acute intrinsic renal failure in cats: 32 cases (1997–2004). J Am Vet Med Assoc 2008;232(5):728–32.

23. Uchino S. Acute renal failure in critically Ill patients: a multinational, multicenter study. JAMA 2005;294(7):813–8.

24. Behrend EN, Grauer GF, Mani I, et al. Hospital-acquired acute renal failure in dogs: 29 cases (1983–1992). J Am Vet Med Assoc 1996;208(4):537–41.

25. Kenney EM, Rozanski EA, Rush JE, et al. Association between outcome and organ system dysfunction in dogs with sepsis: 114 cases (2003–2007). J Am Vet Med Assoc 2010;236(1):83–7.

26. Brochard L, Abroug F, Brenner M, et al. An official ATS/ERS/ESICM/SCCM/SRLF statement: prevention and management of acute renal failure in the ICU patient: an international consensus conference in intensive care medicine. Am J Respir Crit Care Med 2010;181(10):1128–55.

27. Albarellos G, Montoya L, Ambros L, et al. Multiple once-daily dose pharmacokinetics and renal safety of gentamicin in dogs. J Vet Pharmacol Ther 2004;27(1): 21–5.

28. Grauer GF. Early detection of renal damage and disease in dogs and cats. Vet Clin North Am Small Anim Pract 2005;35(3):581–96.

29. Greco DS, Turnwald GH, Adams R, et al. Urinary gamma-glutamyl transpeptidase activity in dogs with gentamicin-induced nephrotoxicity. Am J Vet Res 1985;46(11):2332–5.

30. Waldrop JE. Urinary electrolytes, solutes, and osmolality. Vet Clin North Am Small Anim Pract 2008;38(3):503–12, ix.

31. Clemo FA. Urinary enzyme evaluation of nephrotoxicity in the dog. Toxicol Pathol 1998;26(1):29–32.

32. Grauer GF, Greco DS, Behrend EN, et al. Effects of dietary protein conditioning on gentamicin-induced nephrotoxicosis in healthy male dogs. Am J Vet Res 1994;55(1):90–7.

33. Grauer GF, Greco DS, Behrend EN, et al. Estimation of quantitative enzymuria in dogs with gentamicin-induced nephrotoxicosis using urine enzyme/creatinine ratios from spot urine samples. J Vet Intern Med 1995;9(5): 324–7.

34. Rivers BJ, Walter PA, O'Brien TD, et al. Evaluation of urine gamma-glutamyl transpeptidase-to-creatinine ratio as a diagnostic tool in an experimental model of aminoglycoside-induced acute renal failure in the dog. J Am Anim Hosp Assoc 1996;32(4):323–36.

35. Maddens BE, Daminet S, Demeyere K, et al. Validation of immunoassays for the candidate renal markers C-reactive protein, immunoglobulin G, thromboxane B2 and retinol binding protein in canine urine. Vet Immunol Immunopathol 2010; 134(3–4):259–64.

36. Smets PM, Meyer E, Maddens BE, et al. Urinary markers in healthy young and aged dogs and dogs with chronic kidney disease. J Vet Intern Med 2010; 24(1):65–72.

37. Grauer GF, Greco DS, Behrend EN, et al. Effects of dietary n-3 fatty acid supplementation versus thromboxane synthetase inhibition on gentamicin-induced nephrotoxicosis in healthy male dogs. Am J Vet Res 1996;57(6):948–56.

38. Whittemore JC, Webb CB. Beyond fluid therapy: treating acute renal failure. Compend Contin Educ Pract Vet 2005;27(4):288–98.

39. Mathews KA, Monteith G. Evaluation of adding diltiazem therapy to standard treatment of acute renal failure caused by leptospirosis: 18 dogs (1998–2001). J Vet Emerg Crit Care 2007;17(2):149–58.

40. Simmons JP, Wohl JS, Schwartz DD, et al. Diuretic effects of fenoldopam in healthy cats. J Vet Emerg Crit Care 2006;16(2):96–103.

41. Kellum JA. The use of diuretics and dopamine in acute renal failure: a systematic review of the evidence. Crit Care 1997;1(2):53–9.

42. Kellum JA, J Md. Use of dopamine in acute renal failure: a meta-analysis. Crit Care Med 2001;29(8):1526–31.

43. Bagshaw SM, Delaney A, Haase M, et al. Loop diuretics in the management of acute renal failure: a systematic review and meta-analysis. Crit Care Resusc 2007;9(1):60–8.

44. Acierno MJ, Maeckelbergh V. Continuous renal replacement therapy. Compend Contin Educ Pract Vet 2008;30(5):264–80.

45. Diehl SH, Seshadri R. Use of continuous renal replacement therapy for treatment of dogs and cats with acute or acute-on-chronic renal failure: 33 cases (2002–2006). J Vet Emerg Crit Care 2008;18(4):370–82.

46. Dorval P, Boysen S. Management of acute renal failure in cats using peritoneal dialysis: a retrospective study of six cases (2003–2007). J Feline Med Surg 2009;11(2):107–15.

47. Langston CE. Hemodialysis. In: Bonagura JD, Twedt DC, editors. Kirk's current veterinary therapy XIV. St Louis (MO): Saunders Elsevier; 2009. p. 896–900.

Hepatic Dysfunction

Kelly W. McCord, DVM, MS[a],*, Craig B. Webb, PhD, DVM[b]

KEYWORDS

- Liver - Failure - Antioxidant

Acute liver failure (ALF) is a rare cause of admission to the critical care unit in human hospitals, but the diagnosis carries with it a high mortality rate.[1] Anecdotally, at the Colorado State University Veterinary Teaching Hospital, liver disease (acute and chronic) and acute liver failure appear to account for a significant portion of critical care patients, and hepatic failure is a sequela of multiple organ dysfunction that can be seen in either setting. Viral hepatitis (A, B, and E) is a leading cause of fulminant hepatic failure in humans, but viral infections are rarely appreciated as a cause of liver disease in dogs and cats. On the other hand, drugs (eg, acetaminophen) and toxins (eg, *Amanita* spp mushrooms) are a common cause of ALF recognized in both patient populations. Liver transplantation is not yet a treatment option for veterinary patients, and several aspects of hepatic physiology and function are unique to each species, especially the feline, so one must exercise caution when interpreting the human literature relative to veterinary medicine. This article defines hepatic dysfunction, highlights the most common causes of acute hepatic failure in dogs and cats, outlines the pathophysiology underlying hepatic manifestations of sepsis and shock in the critical care unit, and discusses useful diagnostic techniques, treatment options, and the prognoses for these critical care patients.

HEPATIC DYSFUNCTION: DEFINITION

Fulminant hepatic failure in humans was first defined as a potentially reversible disorder resulting from severe liver injury and including signs of encephalopathy shortly after the onset of symptoms in patients with no prior history of liver disease.[2] This definition has undergone some revision, but continues to highlight the loss of hepatocellular function and the presence of hepatic encephalopathy, jaundice, and coagulopathy, in patients with no preexisting liver disease.[3] Hepatic dysfunction is further defined as altered alanine aminotransferase (ALT) plasma activities and a progressively increasing serum bilirubin concentration (>5 mg/dL).[4] In veterinary

The authors have nothing to disclose.
[a] Small Animal Internal Medicine, Department of Clinical Sciences, James L. Voss Veterinary Teaching Hospital, Colorado State University, 300 West Drake Road, Fort Collins, CO 80523, USA
[b] Department of Clinical Sciences, James L. Voss Veterinary Teaching Hospital, Colorado State University, 300 West Drake Road, Fort Collins, CO 80523, USA
* Corresponding author.
E-mail address: vetmedguy@yahoo.com

doi:10.1016/j.cvsm.2011.04.002
0195-5616/11/$ – see front matter © 2011 Elsevier Inc. All rights reserved.

vetsmall.theclinics.com

medicine, acute hepatic failure has been defined as a sudden loss of greater than 75% of functional hepatic mass.[5] The result is insufficient hepatic parenchyma to maintain synthetic and excretory demands.[6] The biochemical abnormalities and clinical signs associated with acute hepatic failure in dogs and cats include significant elevations in ALT liver enzyme activity and bilirubin concentration, loss of synthetic capabilities, coagulation abnormalities, and signs of hepatic encephalopathy, as seen in humans.

CAUSES OF ACUTE LIVER FAILURE IN DOGS AND CATS

Table 1 summarizes some of the more frequently encountered causes of ALF in veterinary patients. It is not intended to be a complete or exhaustive list. In fact, the list is quite labile; it grows as new drugs are introduced into veterinary practice (eg, carprofen) or a new series of cases identifies a previously unappreciated hepatotoxin (eg, xylitol). At the same time, other causes will wax and wane in prevalence with the advent of specific vaccines and gradual shifts in territorial distribution (eg, leptospirosis).

HEPATIC MANIFESTATIONS OF SEPSIS

Sepsis is characterized by a systemic inflammatory response syndrome (SIRS) in the presence of a known or suspected source of infection. Activation of the patient's immune system in response to the infection can result in several deleterious or even fatal complications, including ALF. Conversely, patients in ALF are at increased risk for infection and the development of sepsis and SIRS. Shock is often a component of the clinical picture on admission, or an imminent consequence of the rapid progression of the septic state. The liver plays a central role in regulating defense, immunologic, and metabolic functions during sepsis, and is a key element in SIRS. The liver is home to the largest collection of macrophages in the body (Kupffer cells) and therefore is crucial to the control of systemic endotoxemia, bacteremia, and vasoactive byproducts. These Kupffer cells are also capable of increased cytokine production and release in response to inflammatory signals or changes in hepatic oxygenation, as well as producing acute-phase proteins that affect metabolism and inflammation early in the course of the patient's response to sepsis.[7] Typically the causative agent in sepsis is the endotoxin lipopolysaccharide (LPS) of gram-negative organisms, but any organism with the ability to activate the complement cascade and a cell-mediated immune response is capable of causing SIRS. When organ function becomes altered secondary to the septic response, a condition known as multiple organ dysfunction syndrome (MODS) occurs. The hallmark of MODS is that physiologic homeostasis cannot be regulated without medical intervention.[4] As reported in the human literature, the likelihood of death increases with an increase in the number of organ systems failing, and patients in which one organ system has failed are more likely to have subsequent systems fail.[4]

In sepsis the initiating cause of hepatic dysfunction can be due to a primary insult to the liver itself, or secondary to an inflammatory stimulus elsewhere in the body. Regardless of the cause, the damage to the liver leads to the clinical signs seen in these patients. Dysfunction of the liver leads to reduced gluconeogenesis and glycolysis, altered protein production and amino acid metabolism, a reduction in the removal of serum triglycerides and, if severe, reduced synthesis of coagulation factors and derangements in host defenses.[8,9] Using an experimental model of sepsis in dogs, it was determined that intracellular glutamine levels are decreased by 41%.[10] Glutamine depletion is likely to occur when there are alterations in protein synthesis as seen with liver dysfunction. Glutamine is necessary to maintain gastrointestinal enterocyte health and function. With a deficit of this amino acid, translocation of gram-negative

Table 1
Causes of acute liver failure in dogs and cats

Category	Specific Example
Drugs	
Anesthetics	Halothane (D)
Antiarrhythmics	Amiodarone (D)
Antibiotics	Potentiated sufonamides (trimethoprim-sulfamethoxazole) (D), nitrofurantoin (D), tetracycline (D, C)
Anticonvulsants	Phenobarbitol (D), oral diazepam (C) , clonazepam (C)
Antifungals	Itraconazole (D, C), ketoconazole (D, C), griseofulvin (C)
Antiparasitic, anthelmintic	Mebendazole
Antithyroid	Methimazole (C)
Chemotherapeutics	Lomustine (CCNU) (D)
Cytotoxic (adrenal gland)	Mitotane (D)
Immunomodulators	Azathioprine (C, D), cyclosporine
NSAIDs, pain medications	Carprofen (Rimadyl) (D), acetaminophen (C, D)
Nutraceuticals	Galactosamine, kava kava (D), comfrey extract
Oral hypoglycemics	Glipizide (C)
Steroids	Stanozolol (C), danazol (D)
Toxins	
Aflatoxins/mycotoxins	*Aspergillus,* moldy foodstuffs, contaminated pet food
Amanita mushrooms	*Amanita phylloides*
Chlorinated hydrocarbons	CCl_4, naphthalenes (moth balls)
Heavy metals	Copper, zinc, iron, mercury
Phenols	Lysol disinfectant (C), pine oil
Plants	Sago palm nuts, Blue-green algae, Cycad palm
Polyol (sugar substitute)	Xylitol
Poison	Phosphorus rat poison
Infectious Agents	
Bacterial, fungal, protozoal	Leptospirosis (D), clostridiosis, histoplasmosis, toxoplasmosis, neosporosis
Endotoxemia	*Clostridium perfringens, Clostridium difficile* endotoxin
Septicemia	*Escherichia coli*
Viral, Rickettsial	Adenovirus I (D), canine herpesvirus (D), FIP (C), *Ehrlichia, Rickettsia rickettsii*
Perfusion and Hypoxia	
	DIC, liver lobe torsion or entrapment, hemolytic anemia
	Hypovolemic shock, circulatory shock, surgical/anesthetic hypotension/hypoxia
	Multiple organ dysfunction syndrome
	Systemic inflammatory response syndrome
	Thromboembolic disease, caval syndrome
Other	
Hyperthermia	Heatstroke
Inflammation	Severe acute pancreatitis, septicemia, endotoxemia
Metabolic, neoplasia	Hepatic lipidosis (C), lymphoma

Abbreviations: C, cats; D, dogs; DIC, disseminated intravascular coagulation; FIP, feline infectious peritonitis; NSAIDs, nonsteroidal anti-inflammatory drugs.

bacteria from the gut may expose the liver to a significantly increased burden of endotoxin.[8,9,11,12] Although the translocation of bacteria itself is not necessarily damaging, in septic patients the proinflammatory response is already activated and minor insults can cause augmented host responses. This "2-hit" theory of MODS is thought to be due to the activation of mononuclear cells with a massive release of cytokines (interleukin [IL]-1β, IL-6, and tumor necrosis factor [TNF]-α) causing an overexaggerated immune response and signs of septic shock.[13,14] A reduction in hepatic oxygenation, as commonly seen in sepsis and MODS, generates reactive oxygen species, which further modulate the release, binding, and cytotoxicity of cytokines, including TNF-α.[15]

Seventy-five percent of the blood flow to the liver arrives through splanchnic venous drainage, with the remaining blood flowing from hepatic arteries. In healthy individuals the two systems remain in balance such that 25% to 30% of cardiac output is brought to the liver.[16] In septic shock, splanchnic venous drainage increases in proportion to the cardiac output while hemoglobin saturation is decreased in the portal blood.[17] Although it would seem that the increased blood flow would prevent hypoxia, this is not always the case. There is likely an increase in oxygen demand with sepsis, and with the increased portal flow there is typically a decrease in hepatic arterial blood flow—a physiologic buffer system that ends up becoming a paradoxic insult to an already compromised organ.

Hypoxemia, cytokine effects, and increased bacterial burden to the liver lead to cytopathology, which is usually characterized by necrosis or apoptosis. One hallmark of acute liver insult and hepatocellular damage is an elevation in the activities of both hepatic transaminase enzymes (ALT and aspartate aminotransferase [AST]). Both are cytosolic enzymes that leak from damaged hepatocytes and are easily detected in the serum. ALT is almost exclusively produced by hepatocytes, whereas AST is produced in other tissues such as muscle and red blood cells. For this reason, elevations in both enzymes are more suggestive of hepatotoxicity (cellular damage or inflammation), as opposed to elevations in AST alone. The degree of elevation does not necessarily correlate with the degree of hepatic dysfunction; significant increases in the serum levels of these enzymes can be seen even with a normally functioning liver. In fact, in cases of chronic hepatic disease in which cirrhosis occurs, the enzyme levels may normalize over time because of the decreased mass of hepatocytes. Therefore, more specific measures of hepatic function are needed to assess the liver's synthetic and metabolic capabilities. Several normal hepatic metabolites and synthetic products can be measured with routine chemistry analyzers; these include glucose, urea, cholesterol, albumin, and coagulation factors. Elevations in total bilirubin indicate hepatic dysfunction if hemolysis and post-hepatic obstructive processes have been ruled out. It is possible for there to be a significant decrease in liver function while still being presented with normal chemistry and coagulation parameters. In these situations, measurement of fasted and postprandial serum bile acids can be a more sensitive combination of tests for determining hepatic function. Additional laboratory abnormalities may be associated with specific diseases causing hepatic dysfunction, and are discussed in other sections of this article.

ASCITES AND ELECTROLYTE ABNORMALITIES AS MANIFESTATIONS OF HEPATIC DYSFUNCTION

With severe hepatic dysfunction a cascade of neurohormonal events leads to changes in vascular compliance, redistribution of blood flow via vasodilatory mechanisms, and altered hormone signaling, which eventually lead to ascites formation. Sinusoidal hypertension likely occurs secondary to architectural changes in the liver parenchyma with distortion of the flow of blood through the sinusoids. Portal hypertension is recognized locally, leading to the appropriate release of vasodilatory mediators such as nitric oxide, endothelin, vasoactive intestinal peptide, glucagon, bile acids, and prostaglandins. Release of these mediators systemically causes vasodilation and redistribution of blood flow to the venous system.[18] Activation of the baroreceptor-mediated renin-angiotensin-aldosterone system (RAAS) ensues and promotes retention of sodium (via aldosterone) and water (via vasopressin). Splanchnic vasodilation also allows for increased and excessive lymphatic flow leading to hepatic capsule leakage of lymphatic fluid and drainage of the fluid into the peritoneum. If there is persistent activation of the systems that allow for water and sodium retention, compensatory renal vasoconstriction can become severe enough to cause functional renal insufficiency, which is known as the hepatorenal syndrome. This functional renal failure occurs as a result of decreased glomerular filtration rate (GFR), not tubular or interstitial damage, and can lead to renal hypoperfusion and permanent renal damage if not addressed. In humans this condition is diagnosed when a precipitous drop in GFR occurs with no other cause of acute renal failure found, renal sodium excretion is impaired (<10 mEq/d), and the osmolality of the urine is found to be greater than the plasma osmolality, all in the presence of hepatic failure.[19]

Hepatic insufficiency can also lead to significant abnormalities in potassium, phosphorus, and magnesium regulation, further leading to specific abnormalities that result in patient complications. Hypokalemia occurs with excessive vomiting or diarrhea, intestinal malabsorption, poor nutrition, activation of the RAAS system, or iatrogenic causes (eg, loop diuretic therapy). Hypokalemia has been documented frequently in cases of canine hepatic cirrhosis with and without ascites, canine portosystemic shunts, and feline hepatic lipidosis.[19] Hypokalemia can lead to worsening signs of hepatic encephalopathy because transcellular shifts between potassium and hydrogen cause a decrease in ammonia clearance by the kidneys. When potassium is low, hydrogen ions enter cells and are unavailable as a titratable acid in the renal tubules for ammonia excretion. Alternatively, when potassium is infused into a hypokalemic patient, potassium enters cells, displacing hydrogen into the plasma, where the hydrogen is then available for excretion into the renal tubular lumen and irreversibly combines with ammonia for elimination of both in the form of an ammonium ion. Hypophosphatemia in patients with hepatic insufficiency most commonly occurs during refeeding syndrome in cats with hepatic lipidosis, usually within the first 48 hours of nutritional supplementation. Clinical signs of hypophosphatemia typically occur when the serum levels drop below 1.5 mg/dL but are life-threatening when below 1 mg/dL.[20] Clinical or laboratory abnormalities associated with hypophosphatemia include severe muscle weakness leading to respiratory failure, red blood cell hemolysis, ileus and vomiting, thrombocytopathias, neurologic signs that can be misinterpreted as hepatic encephalopathy, seizures, and death.[19,20] Hypomagnesemia occurs uncommonly in hepatic insufficiency. Magnesium is an essential coenzyme for mitochondrial function, and deficits likely occur for reasons similar to the transcellular shifting that occurs with potassium and phosphorus. If left untreated, hypomagnesemia can lead to cardiac, neurologic, and musculoskeletal dysfunction.

CENTRAL NERVOUS SYSTEM DYSFUNCTION IN ACUTE LIVER FAILURE

Although electrolytes play a key role in neurologic dysfunction in patients with liver disease, the encephalopathic condition seen with ALF is likely mediated by changes in central nervous system (CNS) levels of ammonia, glutamate, γ-aminobutyric acid, serotonin, and endogenous benzodiazepines. These factors alter the activity of cells of the CNS or damage the neurons themselves, either directly or indirectly. Additional factors leading to neurologic signs might include circulating exogenous toxins, hemorrhage in the CNS secondary to clotting factor or platelet inhibition, hypoglycemia, acute respiratory distress, and other concurrent diseases such as infection, inflammatory conditions, or neoplasia.

Of particular concern in patients with ALF and encephalopathy is the increased plasma ammonia concentrations that lead to cerebral edema. Increased intracranial pressures occur because of glutamine accumulation in astrocytes, increased blood flow to the brain secondary to vasodilation, and release of inflammatory cytokines. Cerebral edema can predispose patients to brain herniation, which is one of the most common causes of death in patients with ALF.[21]

Clinical signs of encephalopathy include changes in mentation, including anything from simple lethargy to being completely comatose, head pressing, aggression or agitation, convulsions, or seizures. With cerebral edema, neurologic signs might also include altered pupillary light reflexes, peripheral weakness, abnormal respirations and, if severe, the Cushing reflex (bradycardia and systemic hypertension), indicating ensuing brain herniation. Treatment of these conditions is discussed in the later section on treatment.

RISK FACTORS FOR HEPATIC DYSFUNCTION AND FAILURE

Causes of liver dysfunction and failure range from exogenous ingested materials such as chemicals, drugs, environmental agents, food additives, and alternative medicines, to acquired diseases such as neoplasia, infections (viral, bacterial, protozoal, parasitic, and fungal), immune-mediated conditions, metabolic diseases, congenital and genetic disorders, and ischemic events (see **Table 1**).

The icteric form of leptospirosis, which is similar to Weil syndrome in humans, causes hepatic, renal, and vascular dysfunction. Although acute renal failure is the more common presentation of infected dogs, hepatic disease is also seen, even as the sole manifestation of the disease. This organism is typically acquired from urine of reservoir hosts and penetrates the mucosal or skin surfaces of dogs. Bacteremia results in vascular damage and invasion of organs and tissues. The hepatic insult is thought to be due to immune-mediated damage and likely depends on the serovar present. The most common biochemical changes are hyperbilirubinemia, elevated alkaline phosphatase (ALP) activity (due to cholestasis of sepsis), and less marked elevations in ALT activity; however, several confirmed cases by the authors have had markedly elevated ALT and AST activities. Concurrent hepatic disease could not be ruled out in these cases, but liver enzymes returned to normal after specific treatment for leptospirosis. Abnormalities associated with this infection may involve thrombocytopenia (30%–50%), vasculitis from endothelial damage, and pulmonary hemorrhage, which manifests on radiographs as whole lung or caudodorsal reticulonodular pulmonary opacities.[22] Other noteworthy pathogens that may cause hepatic dysfunction in dogs are canine adenovirus, ehrlichiosis, salmonellosis, *Rickettsia rickettsii*, *Toxoplasma gondii*, *Neospora caninum*, *Dirofilaria immitis*, systemic mycoses (in particular *Histoplasma* spp), trematode infections (due to hepatic migration), and hepatozoonosis. In cats, feline infectious peritonitis, bacterial infections of the liver, *T gondii*, trematodes, and rarely *Histoplasma* spp are important causes of hepatic dysfunction.

Organic and synthetic hepatotoxins are also common causes of liver damage in veterinary patients (see **Table 1**). Xylitol, a sugar substitute in chewing gum, has been found to cause elevated liver enzymes or liver failure, 8–12 hours postingestion in dogs. Doses of 1.4–2.0 g/kg have been reported to cause hepatic necrosis.[23] Acetaminophen has been one of the most commonly documented causes of ALF in humans. Cats are particularly sensitive to the metabolite of this drug, known as N-acetyl-p-benzoquinoneimine (NAPQI), because of the limited ability of the feline liver to perform phase I conjugation, which occurs even with very small doses in this species. When phase II hepatic enzymes are overwhelmed, the compound cannot be excreted by the kidneys. The drug is then converted to NAPQI, which causes hepatocellular necrosis by binding to cell proteins.[21] The consequences of this reaction are of particular concern when significant hepatic oxidative stress is present, as glutathione antioxidant reserves are depleted and cannot conjugate the toxic metabolite for excretion from the body. Carprofen was implicated in idiosyncratic acute hepatotoxicity in a case series of 21 dogs.[24] The proposed mechanism of this reaction is immune-mediated destruction of hepatocytes, but has not been fully elucidated. Labrador retrievers seem to be predisposed, and the case series reported a mortality rate of 20%.

The specific cause of ALF from hepatotoxicants cannot be elucidated from biopsy samples, biochemical analyses, or from the clinical signs, because by the time the damage to the liver occurs, the drug or compound has typically been eliminated from or transformed in the body. For other acquired forms of liver dysfunction there is a much greater chance that the underlying etiology can be determined with clinical investigation. Particular examples include neoplasia, infections, and metabolic disturbances (eg, hepatic lipidosis in cats, and congenital and acquired copper storage disease in dogs). Unfortunately, many patients who are presented to the critical care unit with ALF are not stable enough to undergo liver biopsy. If neoplasia, an immune-mediated disease, a metabolic disorder, or an infection is suspected, a biopsy can be extremely useful and may make the difference between a meaningful recovery or death.

INDICATORS AND DIAGNOSIS OF HEPATIC DYSFUNCTION

It is extremely important for the clinician to remember that elevated liver enzyme activities do not necessarily imply hepatic dysfunction. The aminotransferases, if elevated in the serum, indicate hapatocellular damage, but not hepatic dysfunction per se. Elevated serum levels of the inducible liver enzymes ALP and γ-glutamyltransferase together imply cholestasis, either intrahepatic or post-hepatic. Increases in activities of both of these enzymes can also be induced by other nonhepatic diseases and drugs (eg, glucocorticoids and anticonvulsants). To determine hepatic function, a thorough physical examination along with additional biochemical testing is needed. Physical findings of hepatic failure might include icterus of the sclera, pinnae, or mucous membranes; ascites; edema; a large or small liver; polyuria/polydipsia; abdominal discomfort on palpation; neurologic signs suggestive of hepatic encephalopathy; and other nonspecific signs such as lethargy, poor appetite, diarrhea, vomiting, and weakness. Patients with severe liver dysfunction can present with many, some, or none of these findings. Biochemical changes may be the only indication of disease, especially with subacute or more chronic compensated conditions.

Biochemical indicators of hepatic dysfunction include those products produced by the liver, such as glucose, albumin, cholesterol, and blood urea. The progression of the disease can sometimes be monitored by the step-wise decreases in these factors, based on their individual half-lives. For example, in fulminate ALF, glucose and blood urea may appear low before albumin does, because the former are produced or metabolized immediately, unlike the latter which has a half-life of 2 to 3 weeks in circulation. Typically with acute hepatic necrosis, the leakage enzymes will increase first, followed by increases in total bilirubin, then decreases in clotting factors, then blood urea nitrogen (BUN) and glucose, and finally albumin in the most advanced end stages. With chronic long-standing disease in which cirrhosis is occurring, albumin may start to decrease before glucose, BUN, and clotting factors. It is not until the end stages of chronic disease when there is no hepatic mass in reserve that the decreased synthesis of these products is evident on laboratory tests.

The most sensitive and specific determinant for hepatobiliary dysfunction is an elevation in preprandial and postprandial serum bile acids. There are multiple causes for an elevation in bile acids, including deviations of portal blood flow to the systemic circulation such as with portosystemic shunts and cirrhosis; decreased uptake of bile acids directly by the hepatocytes as seen with necrosis, inflammation, and steroid hepatopathies; cholestasis; and intestinal obstruction in which the bile acids cannot be excreted normally into the duodenum and then taken up in the ileum for portal, then systemic, circulation. Maltese dogs may have elevated bile acids despite having no identifiable hepatobiliary disease.[25] There is no competitive uptake of bilirubin and bile acids by hepatocytes, so it is possible that there can be a peripheral hyperbilirubinemia and normal bile acids with hemolytic disease. If both hemolysis and liver dysfunction are suspected in a patient, performing a serum bile acids test in the face of hyperbilirubinemia may be helpful in ruling out hepatic dysfunction. If hemolysis is not present and there is a hyperbilirubinemia, a bile acids test will be elevated and is redundant. A preprandial bile acids sample that is higher than the postprandial sample can occur when there is spontaneous emptying of the gall bladder during the fasting period, just before collecting the preprandial sample. Causes of low serum bile acids include delayed postprandial gastric emptying, prolonged intestinal transit time in which delivery of the bile acids to the ileum is delayed, and disease of the ileum which results in malabsorption of the bile acids into the portal system. Preprandial bile acid levels above 20 μg/L and postprandial levels above 25 μg/L are very specific for liver disease.[26] An important aspect of bile acids testing is that there is very little correlation between the level of serum bile acids and the degree of histologic lesions or degree of portosystemic shunting, if present. A bile acids test is either normal or abnormal, and does not indicate a specific underlying disease process. The test is, however, very specific for hepatobiliary disease (80% in cats if postprandial bile acids are >20 μg/L, 100% in dogs if >25 μg/L). However, serum bile acids should not be used alone to screen for hepatic function, as they are only moderately sensitive (54%–74%).[25,27]

Other potentially useful hepatic function tests include urinary bile acids, serum ammonium levels, and the ammonia tolerance test. Urinary bile acids are excreted in urine produced during the time serum bile acids are elevated. This test has been shown to be specific for hepatobiliary disease in dogs but is not as sensitive as bile acids testing.[28] In cats, urinary bile acids sensitivity and specificity (87% and 88%, respectively) are similar to those of serum bile acids in this species.[29] Ammonium levels can be measured and, if greater than 46 μmol/L, are very sensitive (98%) and specific (89%) for detecting portovascular anomalies in dogs.[30] However, ammonia is very unstable and requires special handling. The ammonium tolerance test is performed when serum ammonia levels are normal and a portosystemic shunt is suspected. Dogs with already-elevated serum ammonia levels should not have this test performed, as the ammonia levels may exceed a tolerable dose.

Additional diagnostic tests may include abdominal ultrasonography, transcolonic pertechnate scintigraphy, and transplenic portal scintigraphy. Ultrasonography can elucidate architectural abnormalities such as masses, abscesses, and size changes, and also reveal perihepatic abnormalities such as biliary, pancreatic, and peritoneal (ascites) involvement. Transcolonic pertechnate scintigraphy can be useful for finding portosystemic shunts, although transplenic portal scintigraphy is more sensitive for finding portovascular anomalies because the dose is concentrated in a smaller area (administered from a syringe via ultrasound-guided placement of a needle into the splenic parenchyma), and more reliably highlights the portal and splenic veins. However, this technique can miss shunts that begin caudal to the splenic vein.[27]

Magnetic resonance imaging (MRI) and computed tomography are typically used for liver disease in veterinary patients when planning for radiation therapy or for trying to determine the location of portovascular shunts. Studies are currently under way to determine whether differentiating benign from malignant neoplastic processes is possible with MRI.

The gold-standard test for hepatic parenchymal disease (primary and acquired), neoplasia, and microvascular dysplasia (primary portal vein hypoplasia) is biopsy of the tissue. Careful assessment of the patient's ability to coagulate normally is recommended before biopsy. Evaluation of the secondary coagulation system can be ascertained by performing an activated coagulation time, or prothrombin time and activated partial thromboplastin time. The primary coagulation system should also be evaluated by performing a buccal mucosal bleeding time, which is normally less than 5 minutes for small animal patients. Although ultrasound-guided biopsies are sometimes useful and the only means by which some clients may allow the clinician to obtain tissue, they frequently do not yield enough tissue to make an accurate assessment of the hepatic disorder. Either surgical acquisition or laparoscopic biopsy is the preferred route to obtain quality samples for histopathologic evaluation, as well as tissue for culture, metal analysis, and special staining, if indicated. Postbiopsy gross visualization of the biopsy sites is also important to make sure excessive hemorrhage is controlled; this is difficult to assess with ultrasonography.

TREATMENT OF LIVER DYSFUNCTION

The specific treatments for the multitude of hepatic diseases that may result in admission to the critical care unit are beyond the scope of this article. However, the goals of treatment and antioxidant treatments for liver disease are briefly discussed. **Table 2** lists treatments specific to hepatic encephalopathy with or without cerebral edema. See **Table 3** for the treatment of complications secondary to liver failure.

The goals of treating liver disease are to identify and eliminate the cause of the insult, support hepatocellular regeneration and prevent further oxidative damage, and manage multisystemic complications of organ failure. A thorough assessment of the patient's ability to coagulate blood properly and maintain a normoglycemic state, a normal blood pressure, and a normal electrolyte and acid-base status are essential in order for the clinician to determine whether the homeostatic control mechanisms of the body and liver are functional. If not, medical intervention is required and the patient should be hospitalized. The secondary systemic effects of liver failure can be life-threatening in themselves, and special attention must be paid to these issues while also addressing the liver itself. There are multiple excellent reviews on treating these conditions.[18,20,30]

For primary hepatic support, the authors recommend the use of antioxidant therapy until the underlying disease is eliminated or placed in remission. If neither can be achieved, continued use of these supplements is indicated. S-Adenosylmethionine (SAMe) is an enzyme in the transsulfuration, transmethylation, and aminopropylation

Table 2
Treatment of hepatic encephalopathy (cerebral edema) in dogs and cats

Drug	Mechanism of Action	Dose
Lactulose	Metabolized into acids that lower the colonic pH and convert ammonia into ammonium, which cannot be absorbed systemically. Also alters bacterial metabolism to reduce bacterial toxins	0.25–0.5 mL/kg PO every 6–8 h until stools are loose. 1–10 mL/kg (3 parts lactulose, 7 parts warm water) as retention enema for 20–30 min. Measure post-enema fluid pH and repeat if >6.0
Metronidazole	Alters colonic bacterial flora to reduce ammonia production	7.5 mg/kg PO every 8–12 h
Neomycin	Poorly systemically absorbed; alters colonic bacterial flora to reduce ammonia production	22 mg/kg PO every 8 h
Mannitol	Increases vascular osmotic pressures and helps retain fluids intravascularly	0.5 g/kg IV over 15 min
Flumazenil	Short-acting benzodiazepine antagonist	0.01–0.02 mg/kg IV as needed

Abbreviations: IV, intravenous; PO, by mouth.

pathways. Glutathione, the most abundant antioxidant in mammalian cells, is produced from the transsulfuration pathway and is frequently decreased in liver disease, although it cannot be supplemented directly. Glutathione is a crucial component of the liver's ability to deal with reactive oxidative species and metabolites from the hepatic processing of toxins, drugs, and xenobiotics, and studies have shown an increase in hepatic

Table 3
Treatment of complications secondary to liver failure in dogs and cats

Condition	Treatment	Dose
Coagulopathies	Fresh-frozen plasma	5–20 mL/kg over 4 h
	Vitamin K$_1$	0.5–1 mg/kg IM or SC once daily for 3 days
GI Ulceration	Sucralfate	Dogs: 0.5–1 g every 8 h in water as slurry before feeding. Cats: 0.25–0.5 g every 8 h as slurry
	Omeprazole	0.7 mg/kg PO once daily
	Famotidine	0.5–1 mg/kg PO, SC, IV once daily
Hypoglycemia	Dextrose (25%)	2–10 mL IV over 10 min
Acute renal failure	Furosemide	Dogs: 2–4 mg/kg IV bolus. Cats: 1–2 mg/kg IV bolus. Follow with 1 mg/kg/h CRI
	Mannitol	0.5–1 g/kg IV over 10–15 min
	Dopamine	1–5 μg/kg/min CRI
Electrolyte abnormalities	KCl	Do not exceed 0.5 mEq/kg/h
	MgCl for hypomagnesemia	1 mEq/kg/d for first day; then 0.5–0.75 mEq/kg/d thereafter
	Sodium phosphates or potassium phosphates	0.03–0.06 mmol/kg/h

Abbreviations: CRI, continuous rate infusion; GI, gastrointestinal; IM, intramuscular; IV, intravenous; PO, by mouth; SC, subcutaneous.

glutathione content following SAMe supplementation. The supplement should be administered on an empty stomach to facilitate bioavailability. A recommended dose of SAMe is 20 mg/kg daily in dogs and cats.

Milk thistle (silymarin) is a flavonolignan isomer that has antioxidant and free-radical scavenging properties. In humans it is used to treat alcoholic liver cirrhosis, viral diseases, and acetaminophen and other toxicities. Milk thistle has been used successfully in the management of people with *Amanita* spp mushroom toxicity. This drug is administered intravenously to humans with this condition, and is particularly useful in preventing hepatic damage from the toxin in this fungus.[31] Many oral formulations of this product are available. It is important to remember that silybin, the isomer of silymarin that comprises the majority of the flavonolignan in the milk thistle plant, is the most bioactive isomer but is found in varying concentrations in each product. There has been no consensus reached as to the proper dose of this compound in humans or veterinary patients. A commercial product is available for dogs and cats that is bound to phosphatidylcholine, which helps improve intestinal absorption (Marin; Nutramax Laboratories, Inc, Edgewood, MD, USA) with a proposed dose range of 5 to 10 mg/kg daily in dogs and cats. An intravenous form called silibinin dihemisuccinate can be administered for *Amanita* mushroom toxicity at a recommended dose of 5 mg/kg over 1 hour, then 70 mg/kg every 12 hours.[21]

Vitamin E is a fat-soluble vitamin that relies on bile acids and pancreatic fluids for maximal absorption. Vitamin E is particularly well suited to break the chain of cell membrane lipid peroxidation that results from excessive oxidative stress. When given at high dosages, however, it can compete with other fat-soluble vitamins such as vitamin K and lead to coagulopathies. Therefore, although this compound is a proven antioxidant and is commonly dosed at 10 mg/kg daily, if a vitamin K–deficient coagulopathy is suspected, vitamin E should not be used.[32]

N-Acetylcysteine increases mitochondrial and cytosolic concentrations of glutathione in hepatocytes, and has been proven as an antidote in humans for acetaminophen poisoning and ALF associated with this condition. Since the 1970s this drug has been shown to prevent liver failure in patients with this toxicity by replacing glutathione levels if administered within the first 8 to 10 hours after ingestion or overdose. The drug has been shown to have free-radical scavenging, hemodynamic, and cytokine effects.[33–35] However, it has also recently been shown in a murine model that use of this medication at doses used in humans and veterinary patients inhibits liver regeneration by activating nuclear factor κB, an effect that is more pronounced when administered long term.[36] Current recommendations for doses come from the human literature and some feline and porcine studies, in which administration of this compound caused improvement of mean arterial pressures, a restoration of vascular endothelial responsiveness to nitric oxide including improved microcirculatory blood flow, and cytoprotective properties for endothelial cells.[37–39] The previously recommended dose was intravenous administration of 140 mg/kg given first, followed by 70 mg/kg every 6 hours for 7 total treatments. The murine model previously discussed revealed that the impaired liver regenerative capacity was more pronounced at 72 hours than at 24 hours, which may preclude using this product for the currently recommended length of time.

Many formulations of these medications are available for enteral administration only. This issue can be of particular concern for patients with active vomiting. In the hospital setting, vomiting can typically be controlled with an arsenal of intravenous or other injectable medications, which may facilitate administration of orally administered hepatoprotectants. If vomiting cannot be well controlled, the medications intended for intravenous administration may be the only option.

PROGNOSIS

The prognosis for ALF is highly variable and depends on the stage of disease, the cause, and the response to treatment. Negative prognostic factors found in humans include elevated prothrombin time, severe hyperbilirubinemia, persistent acidemia, persistent hypernatremia, and cerebral edema.[37] Although these factors are assumed to be similar for veterinary patients, to the best of the authors' knowledge they have not been published.

SUMMARY

Whether severe hepatic dysfunction and ALF occur independent of any other illness, occur as sequelae of sepsis, SIRS, and MODS, or occur and contribute to the subsequent development of sepsis, all scenarios result in a critically ill patient that must be addressed early, aggressively, and with insight into the tremendous number of variables that will ultimately affect the successful management of the potentially fatal set of circumstances.

REFERENCES

1. Bernal W, Auzinger G, Dhawan A, et al. Acute liver failure. Lancet 2010; 376(9736):190–201.
2. Trey C, Davidson CS. The management of fulminant hepatic failure. Prog Liver Dis 1970;3:282–98.
3. Craig DG, Lee A, Hayes PC, et al. The current management of acute liver failure. Aliment Pharmacol Ther 2010;31(3):345–58.
4. Johnson V, Gaynor A, Chan DL, et al. Multiple organ dysfunction syndrome in humans and dogs. J Vet Emerg Crit Care 2004;14(3):158–66.
5. Guilford WG, Center SA, Strombeck DR, et al. Acute hepatic injury: hepatic necrosis and fulminant hepatic failure. In: Center SA, editor. Strombeck's small animal gastroenterology. 3rd edition. Philadelphia: Saunders; 1996. p. 654–704.
6. Hughes D, King LG. The diagnosis and management of acute liver failure in dogs and cats. Vet Clin North Am Small Anim Pract 1995;25(2):437–60.
7. Matuschak GM. Lung-liver interactions in sepsis and multiple organ failure syndrome. Clin Chest Med 1996;17(1):83–98.
8. Mizock BA. Metabolic derangements in sepsis and septic shock. Crit Care Clin 2000;16(2):319–36, vii.
9. Druml W, Heinzel G, Kleinberger G. Amino acid kinetics in patients with sepsis. Am J Clin Nutr 2001;73(5):908–13.
10. Karner J, Roth E, Ollenschlager G, et al. Glutamine-containing dipeptides as infusion substrates in the septic state. Surgery 1989;106(5):893–900.
11. Novak F, Heyland DK, Avenell A, et al. Glutamine supplementation in serious illness: a systematic review of the evidence. Crit Care Med 2002;30(9):2022–9.
12. Goeters C, Wenn A, Mertes N, et al. Parenteral L-alanyl-L-glutamine improves 6-month outcome in critically ill patients. Crit Care Med 2002;30(9):2032–7.
13. Price SA, Spain DA, Wilson MA, et al. Altered vasoconstrictor and dilator responses after a "two-hit" model of sequential hemorrhage and bacteremia. J Surg Res 1999; 81(1):59–64.
14. Garrison RN, Spain DA, Wilson MA, et al. Microvascular changes explain the "two-hit" theory of multiple organ failure. Ann Surg 1998;227(6):851–60.
15. Chaudhri G, Clark IA. Reactive oxygen species facilitate the in vitro and in vivo lipopolysaccharide-induced release of tumor necrosis factor. J Immunol 1989; 143(4):1290–4.

16. Dahn MS, Lange P, Lobdell K, et al. Splanchnic and total body oxygen consumption differences in septic and injured patients. Surgery 1987;101(1):69–80.

17. Meier-Hellmann A, Specht M, Hannemann L, et al. Splanchnic blood flow is greater in septic shock treated with norepinephrine than in severe sepsis. Intensive Care Med 1996;22(12):1354–9.

18. Kashani A, Landaverde C, Medici V, et al. Fluid retention in cirrhosis: pathophysiology and management. QJM 2008;101(2):71–85.

19. Center SA. Fluid, electrolyte, and acid-base disorders in liver disease. In: DiBartola SP, editor. Fluid, electrolyte, and acid-base disorders in small animal practice. 3rd edition. St Louis (MO): Saunders Elsevier; 2006. p. 437–77.

20. Schenck PA. Electrolyte disorders: Ca-P and Mg. In: Ettinger S, Feldman EC, editors. Textbook of veterinary internal medicine diseases of the dog and the cat, vol. 1. 7th edition. St Louis (MO): Saunders Elsevier; 2010. p. 308–14.

21. Cooper J, Webster C, Colahan P, et al. Acute liver failure. Compendium 2006; 28(7):498–514.

22. Baumann D, Fluckiger M. Radiographic findings in the thorax of dogs with leptospiral infection. Vet Radiol Ultrasound 2001;42(4):305–7.

23. Todd JM, Powell LL. Xylitol intoxication associated with fulminant hepatic failure in a dog. J Vet Emerg Crit Care 2007;17(3):286–9.

24. MacPhail CM, Lappin MR, Meyer DJ, et al. Hepatocellular toxicosis associated with administration of carprofen in 21 dogs. J Am Vet Med Assoc 1998;212(12): 1895–901.

25. Webster CR. History, clinical signs, and physical findings in hepatobiliary disease. In: Ettinger S, Feldman EC, editors. Textbook of veterinary internal medicine diseases of the dog and the cat, vol. 2. 7th edition. St Louis (MO): Saunders Elsevier; 2010. p. 1612–25.

26. Thrall MA, Baker DC, Campbell TW, et al. Laboratory evaluation of the liver. In: Thrall MA, editor. Veterinary hematology and clinical chemistry. Baltimore (MD): Lippincott Williams & Wilkins; 2004. p. 355–75.

27. Webster CR, Cooper JC. Diagnostic approach to hepatobiliary disease. In: Bonagura JD, Twedt DC, editors. Kirk's current veterinary therapy XIV. St Louis (MO): Saunders Elsevier; 2009. p. 543–9.

28. Balkman CE, Center SA, Randolph JF, et al. Evaluation of urine sulfated and nonsulfated bile acids as a diagnostic test for liver disease in dogs. J Am Vet Med Assoc 2003;222(10):1368–75.

29. Trainor D, Center SA, Randolph F, et al. Urine sulfated and nonsulfated bile acids as a diagnostic test for liver disease in cats. J Vet Intern Med 2003;17(2):145–53.

30. Gerritzen-Bruning MJ, van den Ingh TS, Rothuizen J. Diagnostic value of fasting plasma ammonia and bile acid concentrations in the identification of portosystemic shunting in dogs. J Vet Intern Med 2006;20(1):13–9.

31. Seeff LB, Lindsay KL, Bacon BR, et al. Complementary and alternative medicine in chronic liver disease. Hepatology 2001;34(3):595–603.

32. Flatland B. Hepatic support therapy. In: Bonagura JD, Twedt DC, editors. Kirk's current veterinary therapy XIV. St Louis (MO): Saunders Elsevier; 2009. p. 555–7.

33. Yang R, Miki K, He X, et al. Prolonged treatment with N-acetylcysteine delays liver recovery from acetaminophen hepatotoxicity. Crit Care 2009;13(2):R55.

34. Dambach DM, Durham SK, Laskin JD, et al. Distinct roles of NF-kappaB p50 in the regulation of acetaminophen-induced inflammatory mediator production and hepatotoxicity. Toxicol Appl Pharmacol 2006;211(2):157–65.

35. Adamson GM, Harman AW. Oxidative stress in cultured hepatocytes exposed to acetaminophen. Biochem Pharmacol 1993;45(11):2289–94.

36. Prescott LF, Park J, Ballantyne A, et al. Treatment of paracetamol (acetaminophen) poisoning with N-acetylcysteine. Lancet 1977;2(8035):432–4.

37. Polson J, Lee WM. AASLD position paper: the management of acute liver failure. Hepatology 2005;41(5):1179–97.

38. Dempsey RJ, Kindt GW. Experimental acute hepatic encephalopathy: relationship of pathological cerebral vasodilation to increased intracranial pressure. Neurosurgery 1982;10(6 Pt 1):737–41.

39. Ytrebo LM, Korvald C, Nedredal GI, et al. N-acetylcysteine increases cerebral perfusion pressure in pigs with fulminant hepatic failure. Crit Care Med 2001; 29(10):1989–95.

Gastrointestinal Complications of Critical Illness in Small Animals

Timothy B. Hackett, DVM, MS

KEYWORDS

- MODS • Systemic inflammatory response syndrome • Sepsis
- Bacterial translocation • Arginine • Glutamine

After ingestion, the gastrointestinal (GI) tract stores, propels, mixes, and digests food; secretes enzymes and fluids; and selectively absorbs water, electrolytes, and nutrients. Enormous quantities of fluids and electrolytes are cycled through the intestine each day. Almost half of the total volume of extracellular fluid is secreted in the upper GI tract daily, an amount that greatly exceeds normal intake; yet loss of fecal water and electrolytes is less than 0.1% of the fluid cycled through the GI tract.[1,2] With abnormal secretion and/or impaired absorption, the potential for massive fluid and electrolyte imbalances exists.

The GI tract and liver are considered the shock organs of dogs.[1] GI dysfunction can accompany sepsis, and the systemic inflammatory response syndrome in patients with multiple organ dysfunction syndrome (MODS). The GI tract is subject to damage from a variety of systemic diseases and is commonly affected by MODS in veterinary patients.[3]

Symptoms of GI dysfunction, commonly seen in states of shock, cover a wide clinical spectrum from mild changes in appetite to serious loss of intestinal mucosal integrity, hemorrhagic diarrhea, enteric bacterial translocation, septicemia, and death. GI dysfunction can occur after any cause of tissue hypoxia, poor perfusion and impaired oxygen delivery, because organs supplied by the splanchnic circulation are particularly vulnerable to hypoxia.[4] This response is evident in the hemorrhagic models of shock in which splanchnic perfusion decreases rapidly and disproportionately to other major organ systems.[3]

Although the renal system has azotemia and oliguria to document dysfunction and the central nervous system has a more complex scoring system, the Glasgow Coma Score, to objectively define functional impairment,[5] the GI tract has many functions

The author has nothing to disclose.
Department of Clinical Sciences, Colorado State University, 300 West Drake Road, Fort Collins, CO 80523, USA
E-mail address: Tim.Hackett@colostate.edu

Vet Clin Small Anim 41 (2011) 759–766
doi:10.1016/j.cvsm.2011.05.013   vetsmall.theclinics.com

that are not subject to objective measurements, rendering dysfunction and failure of this system difficult to quantitate. The gut is not just for digestion and nutrient absorption but is a metabolically active, immunologically unique reservoir of potential pathogens.[4] However clinically difficult it may be to monitor splanchnic perfusion, the clinician must remain diligent and attempt to diminish the risk of complications associated with GI dysfunction. Treatment needs to be aggressive and focused on the underlying cause, generally supporting the patient by replacing lost fluids and proteins. Clinicians must also provide nutrition to the GI tract as it heals, all while attempting to prevent the translocation of pathogenic GI flora into the bloodstream.

GI DEFENSE MECHANISMS

Natural defenses against microbial invasion of the gut include the epithelial cell barrier, mucus, gastric acid, pancreatic enzymes, bile, and bowel motility. Structurally, the intestine is a single-layered columnar epithelium arranged in villi and crypts. Cell-to-cell junctional complexes offer selective permeability through tight junctions; maintain intercellular adhesion through intermediate junctions and desmosomes; and allow intercellular communication through gap junctions to control the movement of ions, fluids, and small hydrophilic uncharged compounds, including bacteria and lipopolysaccharides.[6] Mucins, secreted by epithelial goblet cells, hamper bacterial penetration and act as a lubricant to reduce mucosal abrasion and damage induced by acid and other luminal toxins.[7] Mucosal secretions are rich in IgA antibodies that effectively bind bacteria, preventing mucosal adherence and colonization.[8] Bile is another important barrier normally limiting enteric bacterial growth and translocation from the intestine.[9]

BACTERIAL TRANSLOCATION

Bacterial translocation was defined in 1979 as the passage of both viable and nonviable microbes and microbial products, such as endotoxin, from the intestinal lumen through the epithelial mucosa into the mesenteric lymph nodes and other organs.[10] Bacterial translocation can be caused by impaired host defenses, altered GI flora resulting in bacterial overgrowth, physical disruption of the gut mucosal barrier, direct injury to the enterocytes (eg, by irradiation or toxins), or reduced blood flow to the intestine.[11]

The oxygen tension at the tip of the intestinal villus is much lower than that in arterial blood, even under normal conditions; consequently, the susceptibility of the epithelium to hypoxic injury is increased.[11] Any reduction in blood flow aggravates these conditions, and epithelial cell injury may readily develop when the oxygenation of tissues is diminished. In animals with trauma and hemorrhagic, cardiogenic, and septic shock, there is diminished blood flow to the mucosa and submucosa of the jejunum, ileum, and colon, whereas flow to other organs is preserved. Ischemia-induced epithelial injury in the gut is a pathway common to shock and trauma, and this pathway may lead to dysfunction of the gut barrier and set the stage for bacterial translocation.[11] Increased intestinal permeability has been observed in patients with burns,[12] those who underwent elective or emergency surgery,[13] those with hemorrhagic shock,[14] and those with trauma and in intensive care.[15,16]

HEMORRHAGIC DIARRHEA

Acute hemorrhagic diarrhea is one of the most serious clinical manifestations of GI failure faced by small animal practitioners.[17] Diarrhea can cause massive loss of fluids, electrolytes, and proteins. Hemorrhagic diarrhea, regardless of the cause, is the clinical sign of a loss of mucosal integrity. With the loss of this barrier, enteric flora can enter the bloodstream, leading to septicemia. The combination of dehydration, anemia, hypoproteinemia, and septicemia reduces systemic perfusion and oxygen delivery, putting the patient at risk for MODS.[4] Diarrhea results from accumulation of osmotically active particles in the intestinal tract, excess solute secretion, impaired absorption, or alterations in intestinal motility. All these mechanisms should be reviewed because 1 or all may occur together in the individual patient with diarrhea.[1,17]

Osmotic diarrhea results when unabsorbable solutes increase the fecal water content. Osmotic diarrhea can result from overeating, sudden dietary changes, maldigestion, or malabsorption. Some bacterial enterotoxins pathologically enhance secretion. Bacterial pathogens that are known to cause secretory diarrhea include *Escherichia coli*, *Staphylococcus aureus*, *Klebsiella pneumoniae*, *Yersinia enterocolitica*, *Salmonella typhimurium*, *Campylobacter* spp, and *Clostridium perfringens*.[17,18] Enteric hormones, fatty acids, and bile acids also stimulate intestinal secretion. Malabsorption can be caused by anything affecting the mucosal or submucosal layers of the intestine. With damage to the mucosa, normal sodium reabsorption is impaired, fecal water increases, and diarrhea results. Motility changes that speed intestinal transit cause diarrhea. By decreasing transit time, normal water resorption cannot take place and diarrhea results. The most common mechanism of severe hemorrhagic diarrhea is an increase in intestinal permeability.[17]

DIAGNOSTIC EVALUATION

Obtunded dehydrated febrile animals with anorexia, vomiting, and/or diarrhea should be evaluated for concurrent systemic disease and dysfunction of other organ systems. A complete physical examination should identify life-threatening complications associated with loss of blood and fluids. Priority is given to the cardiopulmonary systems. Therapy includes intravenous fluids, supplemental oxygen, electrolyte replacement, and broad-spectrum parenteral antimicrobials. Treatment should commence immediately although a definitive diagnosis is pursued. Severe increases in intestinal permeability are characterized by hypoproteinemia, melena, and hematochezia.[1,4] A complete blood count should always be evaluated. Animals with idiopathic hemorrhagic gastroenteritis may have packed cell volumes as high as 75%. Severe intestinal blood loss can also lead to anemia and panhypoproteinemia. Infection with either *Salmonella* spp or canine parvovirus is associated with neutropenia. Leukocytosis with immature bands is a common finding with systemic infection. Leukocytosis with lymphopenia and eosinopenia (stress leukogram) is a common finding in any debilitated animal with gastroenteritis. A normal leukogram in a sick animal with GI disease should prompt a corticotropin stimulation test to evaluate possible adrenocortical insufficiency.

A complete serum biochemical profile is necessary to evaluate other organ systems. Glucose level should be checked on admission and at least once a day thereafter to detect hypoglycemia associated with sepsis. Concentrations of electrolytes including sodium, chloride, potassium, and magnesium can drop precipitously in anorectic animals with diarrhea. Hyperkalemia with hyponatremia is another indication of adrenocortical insufficiency; however, these changes can also been seen with whipworm (*Trichuris vulpis*) infections. Hypocholesterolemia is another finding with hypoadrenocorticism. Samples to assess baseline renal function, including serum urea nitrogen (BUN), creatinine, phosphorous, calcium, and urine specific gravity, should be collected before intravenous fluid therapy begins.

A fecal examination is indicated in any diarrheic state. In a study, infectious agents were identified in more than 25% of dogs with diarrhea presented to a veterinary teaching hospital.[19] Direct fecal examination should be performed, as should zinc sulfate flotation. Some parasites, *Giardia* spp and *Trichuris*, may be difficult to identify; so multiple examinations or alternative testing modalities should be performed. Acid-fast staining is useful to confirm *Campylobacter jejuni*. Enzyme-linked immunosorbent assays are available to detect canine parvovirus, *Giardia* spp, and *Cryptosporidium parvum* antigens.

Fecal culture is indicated in animals with inflammatory changes on the fecal smear. Pathogenic and zoonotic bacteria causing enterocolitis include *Salmonella* spp, *C jejuni*, *Shigella* spp, and *Y enterocolitica*. The presence of these species of bacteria is of particular concern in hospitalized patients, multi-animal households, kennels, and homes of immunocompromised individuals.[19]

SYMPTOMATIC TREATMENT

The treatment of any medical problem should be based on the primary cause; however, there are numerous serious and predictable systemic complications of acute GI dysfunction that require immediate supportive care. Mild complications may simply require antiemetic therapy and starvation for 12 to 48 hours with a gradual reintroduction of small amounts of an easily digestible diet for several more days.[1] The absence of nutrients in the GI tract reduces secretions and decreases the concentration of osmotically active particles. For this reason, starvation seems a logical step for secretory and osmotic diarrhea. When animals with acute GI disease are starved, the GI tract receives most of its nourishment from the food passing through the bowel. Early feeding of patients with diarrhea may make more sense in those with increased mucosal permeability. Enteral feeding maintains an increase in mucosal barrier integrity and helps minimize malnutrition.[20–22] Human and animal studies have shown that antibacterial host defenses, including lympho-cytes, neutrophils, and gut-associated immune functions, are better preserved in enterally fed humans and animals.[11,21] Enteral nutrition has been linked with the maintenance of intestinal mucosal integrity. In an animal model, starvation and total parenteral nutrition were found to promote bacterial overgrowth, reduce intestinal mucin production, decrease the level of intestinal IgA, cause mucosal atrophy, and accelerate oxidative stress.[21] In critically ill patients, early enteral nutrition reduces septic complications.[11]

FLUID THERAPY

Intravenous fluid therapy is aimed at restoring lost fluids, resolving dehydration, providing normal maintenance requirements, and keeping up with ongoing losses. Oral fluid therapy may be adequate for simple diarrhea in a hydrated animal. Animals with signs of dehydration, hemorrhagic diarrhea, or MODS should have an intravenous catheter placed to receive parenteral fluids and antibiotics. Fluid therapy must be individualized for each patient based on acid-base status, electrolyte concentrations, plasma protein concentrations, and packed cell volume, because these can be highly variable in patients with diarrhea. Choices of which crystalloid fluid to use and the use of whole blood, packed red blood cells, plasma, albumin, or synthetic colloids as required should be based on serial physical examination and monitoring of packed cell volume, serum total solids, and electrolyte concentrations.

ANTIBIOTICS

Normal resident microbial flora of the intestinal tract includes anaerobic bacteria, which outnumber the aerobic gram-negative organisms 100 to 1000 times.[4] The presence of anaerobic flora, which occupies the mucous layer adjacent to the epithelial cells, can prevent the adherence of other potential pathogens. Antibiotic therapy should not simply target the anaerobes. Instead, the clinician should use a balanced approach toward both gram-negative and anaerobic pathogens. The use of antibiotics is controversial with simple diarrhea. However, with severe hemorrhagic diarrhea, the clinician must assume that the patient has a serious loss of intestinal mucosal barrier integrity, and parenteral bactericidal antibiotic therapy is indicated. The goal of antibiotic therapy is to eliminate enteric bacteria that have passed through the mucosa, entered the bloodstream, and occupied the portal and pulmonary circulations. Animals with fecal cultures positive for bacterial pathogens may be treated according to the sensitivity pattern of the culture. Animals with positive blood cultures should have their antibiotic regimen refined based on the organisms identified.

GLUTAMINE, ARGININE, AND OMEGA-3 FATTY ACID SUPPLEMENTATION

Glutamine, arginine, and omega-3 fatty acids have the potential to modulate the activity of the immune system in clinical situations in which altered supply of nutrients exists.[23,24] Enteral diets enhanced with these nutrients have been shown to have significant benefits, including reducing morbidity, mortality, days hospitalized, and septic complications, compared with normal diets.[23,25]

Glutamine is the main metabolic substrate exerting trophic effects on enterocytes, supporting their normal function. Primarily extracted via luminal absorption, adequate glutamine is also synthesized in the normal gut to be considered a nonessential amino acid. However, during states of illness, this synthetic ability is inadequate to meet these metabolic needs of the enterocytes. In these instances, glutamine supplementation may be necessary to form and repair intracellular tight junctions and maintain mucosal integrity. Glutamine is also important in the synthesis of the protective mucous gel layer and is an essential nutrient for proper cellular immune functions.[26] Glutamine metabolism increases in animals with critical illness. Glutamine levels decrease rapidly after injury, and the magnitude of decrease is predictive of mortality in the intensive care unit.[27] Animals can store this important substrate only for 24 to 48 hours. Because glutamine induces stress tolerance and protects against cellular injury, supplementation may prove beneficial in critically ill patients. Dosages for glutamine supplementation have been extrapolated from the human literature. The recommended dosage for dogs with hemorrhagic diarrhea secondary to parvovirus enteritis is 0.5 g/kg/d divided twice a day in drinking water.[28] Several commercial veterinary critical care diets contain added glutamine and arginine.

Arginine level is reduced in patients with trauma and postoperative patients compared with patients with sepsis and controls. This condition is likely because of the increased levels of arginase from activated myeloid cells in these patients.[29] Meta-analysis of human studies evaluating arginine supplementation in nonseptic critically ill patients has shown improved outcomes.[30] Myeloid cells express another enzyme, inducible nitric oxide synthase (iNOS). Unlike in patients with trauma and postoperative patients, patients with sepsis do not have reduced arginine levels. This is probably because, as opposed to arginase, iNOS is predominantly expressed by activated myeloid cells in patients with sepsis.[29] This has potential clinical implications because excess nitric oxide in sepsis may potentiate hypotension and organ dysfunction. In a canine sepsis model, arginine administration was associated with increased plasma arginine; increased nitric oxide products; and worsening shock, organ injury, and mortality rates.[31] The authors concluded that arginine supplementation is not recommended for patients with sepsis.

Omega-3 fatty acid supplementation has been shown to downregulate arginase expression after injury, and like arginine supplementation, omega-3 fatty acid supplementation has been shown to have beneficial outcomes.[32] Fish oil–enriched diets have also been shown to preserve intestinal blood flow and to enhance the host's ability to kill translocated bacteria in various experimental models of bacterial translocation.[33] This effect was attributed to the increased synthesis of vasodilatory prostaglandins, reversing endotoxin-induced intestinal vasoconstriction, enhanced mucous secretion, and downregulated the synthesis of inflammatory cytokines.[34]

ANALGESIC AND ANTIEMETIC THERAPY

Analgesia should be considered in patients showing signs of abdominal pain. Objective serial monitoring of critically ill patients is necessary when pain is appropriately treated. Nonsteroidal and steroidal antiinflammatory drugs may complicate GI hemorrhage by inhibiting the production of normal protective prostaglandins. Narcotic analgesics can be used as long as respiratory and pulmonary functions are monitored and their effects on GI motility considered. Animals with acute inflammation of the GI tract may be extremely nauseous. Nausea may manifest clinically as anorexia, hypersalivation, or emesis. Antiemetic drugs can provide a degree of relief not offered by fluids or analgesics. Maropitant, metoclopramide, ondansetron, dolasetron, and chlorpromazine are all antiemetic drugs available and appropriate for use in veterinary patients.

PROGNOSIS

The prognosis for patients with acute GI dysfunction depends on the etiology and presence of concurrent organ dysfunction. Young dogs with hemorrhagic gastroenteritis syndrome and patient's with hypoadrenocorticism generally respond quickly to volume replacement, and corticosteroid replacement in the case of hypoadrenocorticism, and have an excellent prognosis despite profound bloody diarrhea.[10] Parvoviral enteritis can produce severe dehydration, shock, and multiple organ failure. With aggressive supportive care, mortality rates of 5% to 20% have been reported.[35] Morbidity and mortality for other causes of acute GI hemorrhage depend on the primary cause, presence of bacterial translocation and sepsis, and concurrent organ failure. The challenge to the veterinary clinician is to replace the lost fluids, electrolytes, and proteins while preventing septic complications. It is vital to monitor the major organ function and treat the primary disease and secondary organ dysfunction in a timely manner.

REFERENCES

1. Guilford WG, Strombeck DR. Classification, pathophysiology, and symptomatic treatment of diarrheal diseases. In: Guilford WG, editor. Strombeck's small animal gastroenterology. Philadelphia: W.B. Saunders Company; 1996. p. 351.
2. Kenney EM, Rozanski EA, Rush JE, et al. Association between outcome and organ system dysfunction in dogs with sepsis: 114 cases (2003–2007). J Am Vet Med Assoc 2010;236:83–7.
3. McNeill JR, Stark RD, Greenway CV. Intestinal vasoconstriction after hemorrhage: roles of vasopressin and angiotensin. Am J Physiol 1970;219:1342.

4. Biffl WL, Moore EE. Role of the gut in multiple organ failure. In: Grenvik A, editor. Textbook of critical care. Philadelphia: W.B. Saunders Company; 2000. p. 1627.

5. Teasdale G, Jennett B. Assessment of coma and impaired consciousness. A practical scale. Lancet 1974;2:81–4.

6. Alexander JW, Boyce ST, Babcock GF, et al. The process of microbial translocation. Ann Surg 1990;212:496–510.

7. Aranow JS, Fink MP. Determinants of intestinal barrier failure in critical illness. Br J Anaesth 1996;77:71–81.

8. Spaeth G, Gottwald T, Specian RD, et al. Secretory immunoglobulin A, intestinal mucin, and mucosal permeability in nutritionally induced bacterial translocation in rats. Ann Surg 1994;220:798–808.

9. Wells CL, Jechorek RP, Erlandsen SL. Inhibitory effect of bile on bacterial invasion of enterocytes: possible mechanism for increased translocation associated with obstructive jaundice. Crit Care Med 1995;23:301–7.

10. Berg RD, Garlington AW. Translocation of certain indigenous bacteria from the gastrointestinal tract to the mesenteric lymph nodes and other organs in a gnotobiotic mouse model. Infect Immun 1979;23:403–11.

11. Wiest R, Rath HC. Bacterial translocation in the gut. Best Pract Res Clin Gastroenterol 2003;17:397–425.

12. LeVoyer T, Cioffi WG Jr, Pratt L, et al. Alterations in intestinal permeability after thermal injury. Arch Surg 1992;127:26–9.

13. Roumen RM, van der Vliet JA, Wevers RA, et al. Intestinal permeability is increased after major vascular surgery. J Vasc Surg 1993;17:734–7.

14. Roumen RM, Hendriks T, Wevers RA, et al. Intestinal permeability after severe trauma and hemorrhagic shock is increased without relation to septic complications. Arch Surg 1993;128:453–7.

15. Harris CE, Griffiths RD, Freestone N, et al. Intestinal permeability in the critically ill. Intensive Care Med 1992;18:38–41.

16. Pape HC, Dwenger A, Regel G, et al. Increased gut permeability after multiple trauma. Br J Surg 1994;81:850–2.

17. Dow SW. Acute medical diseases of the small intestine. In: Tams TR, editor. Handbook of small animal gastroenterology. Philadelphia: W.B. Saunders Company; 1996. p. 246–66.

18. Sasaki J, Goryo M, Asahina M, et al. Hemorrhagic enteritis associated with *Clostridium perfringens* type A in a dog. J Vet Med Sci 1999;61:175–7.

19. Hackett TB, Lappin MR. Prevalence of enteric pathogens in dogs. J Vet Intern Med 2003;39:52–6.

20. Deitch EA. Role of the gut in the pathogenesis of sepsis and multiple organ failure. Proceedings, Fifth International Veterinary Emergency and Critical Care Symposium. Madison (WI): Omnipress; 1996. p. 1–4.

21. Alverdy JC, Aoys E, Moss GS. Total parenteral nutrition promotes bacterial translocation from the gut. Surgery 1988;104:185–90.

22. Spaeth G, Specian RD, Berg RD, et al. Bulk prevents bacterial translocation induced by the oral administration of total parenteral nutrition solution. JPEN J Parenter Enteral Nutr 1990;14:442–7.

23. Kudsk KA, Minard G, Croce MA, et al. A randomized trial of isonitrogenous enteral diets after severe trauma. An immune-enhancing diet reduces septic complications. Ann Surg 1996;224:531–40.

24. Calder PC. Immunonutrition may have beneficial effects in surgical patients. BMJ 2003;327:117–8.

25. Jolliet P, Pichard C. Immunonutrition in the critically ill. Intensive Care Med 1999; 25:631–3.
26. Mazzaferro EM, Hackett TB, Wingfield WE, et al. Role of glutamine in health and disease. Compend Contin Educ Pract Vet 2000;22:1094–103.
27. Singleton K, Serkova N, Beckey VE, et al. Glutamine attenuates lung injury and improves survival after sepsis: role of enhanced heat shock protein expression. Crit Care Med 2005;33:1206–13.
28. Macintire DK, Smith-Carr S. Canine parvovirus part II: clinical signs, diagnosis and treatment. Compend Contin Educ Pract Vet 1997;19:291–302.
29. Drover JW, Dhaliwal R, Weitzel L, et al. Perioperative use of arginine-supplemented diets: a systematic review of the evidence. J Am Coll Surg 2011;212:385–99.
30. Wischmeyer PE, Weitzel L, Dhaliwal R, et al. Should peri-operative arginine containing nutrition therapy become routine in the surgical patients? A systematic review of the evidence and meta-analysis. Anesth Analg 2010;110:S-449.
31. Kalil AC, Sevransky JE, Myers DE, et al. Preclinical trial of L-arginine monotherapy alone or with N-acetylcysteine in septic shock. Crit Care Med 2006;34: 2719–28.
32. Bansal V, Ochoa JB, Syres KM, et al. Interactions between fatty acids and arginine metabolism: implications for the design of immune-enhancing diets. JPEN J Parenter Enteral Nutr 2005;29:S75–80.
33. Pscheidl E, Schywalsky M, Tschaikowsky K, et al. Fish oil-supplemented parenteral diets normalize splanchnic blood flow and improve killing of translocated bacteria in a low-dose endotoxin rat model. Crit Care Med 2000;28:1489–96.
34. Denlinger LC. Low-dose prostacyclin reverses endotoxin-induced intestinal vasoconstriction: potential for the prevention of bacterial translocation in early sepsis. Crit Care Med 2001;29:453–4.
35. Prittie J. Canine parvoviral enteritis: a review of diagnosis, management, and prevention. J Vet Emerg Crit Care 2004;14:167–76.

Critical Illness–Related Corticosteroid Insufficiency in Small Animals

Linda G. Martin, DVM, MS[a,b,*]

KEYWORDS

- Relative adrenal insufficiency
- Hypothalamic-pituitary-adrenal axis • Critical illness
- Refractory hypotension
- Sepsis/systemic inflammatory response syndrome • Endocrine

Acute illness can produce dramatic changes in endocrine function.[1–3] Activation of the hypothalamic-pituitary-adrenal (HPA) axis, as evidenced by an increase in secretion of adrenocorticotropin hormone (ACTH) and cortisol during illness, is presumed to be a vital part of the physiologic stress response and is essential for maintenance of homeostasis and adaptation during severe illness. Cortisol has been shown to increase after a variety of stressors, and the response is thought to be proportional to the magnitude of the injury or disease process.[3,4] However, human and animal studies have revealed marked heterogeneity in adrenocortical function in critically ill patients.[5,6]

The syndrome of critical illness–related corticosteroid insufficiency (CIRCI), previously referred to as relative adrenal insufficiency, has been proposed to describe these endocrine abnormalities associated with illness. This syndrome is characterized by an inadequate production of cortisol in relation to an increased demand during periods of severe stress, particularly in critical illnesses such as sepsis or septic shock.[7–9] In patients with CIRCI, cortisol concentrations, despite being normal or high in some patients, may still be inadequate for the current physiologic stress or illness, and the patient is unable to respond to additional stress. CIRCI is usually defined by an inadequate response to exogenous ACTH stimulation.[8,10] This failed response indicates reduced functional integrity of the HPA axis and may lessen the patient's ability to cope with severe illness and stress. In the setting of human and veterinary critical illness, CIRCI appears to be a transient condition secondary to

[a] Department of Clinical Sciences, College of Veterinary Medicine, Auburn University, Auburn, AL 36849, USA
[b] Small Animal Intensive Care Unit, Auburn University Small Animal Teaching Hospital, Auburn, AL, USA
* Department of Clinical Sciences, Hoerlein Hall, Auburn University, AL 36849.
E-mail address: lgm0004@auburn.edu

Vet Clin Small Anim 41 (2011) 767–782
doi:10.1016/j.cvsm.2011.03.021
vetsmall.theclinics.com
0195-5616/11/$ – see front matter © 2011 Elsevier Inc. All rights reserved.

severe illness with adrenal function normalizing after recovery. For these patients, life-long replacement of glucocorticoids is not anticipated.[8,11] This article reviews the physiology and pathophysiology of the corticosteroid response to critical illness and the incidence, clinical features, diagnosis, and treatment of CIRCI.

NORMAL REGULATION OF THE HPA AXIS DURING ILLNESS

Cortisol secretion by the adrenal cortex is under the control of the hypothalamic-pituitary axis. Signals from the body (eg, cytokine release, tissue injury, pain, hypoten-sion, hypoglycemia, and hypoxemia) are sensed by the central nervous system and transmitted to the hypothalamus. The hypothalamus integrates these signals and increases the release of corticotropin-releasing hormone (CRH). CRH circulates to the anterior pituitary gland, in which it stimulates the release of ACTH, which acts on the adrenal cortex stimulating the release of cortisol. Cortisol, released from the adrenal glands or from exogenous sources, feeds back on the HPA axis to inhibit its secretion (negative feedback). Thus, decreased cortisol concentrations (lack of nega-tive feedback) result in increased CRH-ACTH release and conversely elevated cortisol concentrations inhibit CRH-ACTH release. By these mechanisms, the body can control the secretion of cortisol within narrow limits and can respond with increased secretion of cortisol to a variety of stressors and other signals.

Cortisol circulates in the blood in both bound and unbound forms. Almost 90% of cortisol is bound to corticosteroid-binding globulin (CBG). It is the unbound or free cortisol that is physiologically active and homeostatically regulated. Although relative concentrations of free cortisol have not been well investigated in critically ill patients, studies suggest that there is a decrease in cortisol binding rather than an increase.[8,11] The reduced binding results in elevated free cortisol concentrations in the acute phase of illness. The cause for this decrease in binding is unknown, but likely increases cortisol availability to cells and tissues during stress and illness.[8,11]

ABNORMAL RESPONSE OF THE HPA AXIS DURING ILLNESS

The HPA axis, along with the adrenergic and sympathetic nervous systems, is the main mediator of the stress response. During acute illness, circulating proinflamma-tory cytokines, including interleukin (IL)-6, tumor necrosis factor-alpha (TNF-α), and IL-1β, stimulate the production of CRH and ACTH. Simultaneously, vagal afferent fibers detect the presence of cytokines such as IL-1β and TNF-α at the site of inflam-mation and activate the HPA axis. Subsequently, this results in an immediate rise in circulating cortisol concentrations.[12] Cortisol then binds to specific carriers, CBG and albumin, to reach the target tissues. It is generally accepted that CBG-bound cortisol has restricted access to the target cells.[13,14] At the inflammatory sites, elas-tase produced by neutrophils liberates cortisol from CBG, allowing localized delivery of cortisol to the cells.[14] Subsequently, cortisol can freely cross the cell membrane or interact with specific membrane-binding receptor sites. Cytokines may also increase the affinity of receptors for glucocorticoids.[15] Dysfunction at any 1 of these steps can result in diminished cortisol action. Alternately, cortisol can be inactivated by conver-sion to cortisone by 11β-hydroxysteroid dehydrogenase type 2. CIRCI may result from decreased glucocorticoid synthesis or reduced access of glucocorticoids to the target tissues and cells.

Decreased Glucocorticoid Synthesis

Subsequent to the secretion of ACTH, glucocorticoids are synthesized by the adrenal cortex from cholesterol. The amount of glucocorticoid found in adrenal tissue is not sufficient to maintain normal rates of secretion for more than a few minutes in the absence of continuing biosynthesis. Thus, the rate of secretion is directly proportional to the rate of biosynthesis. In other words, any disruption in glucocorticoid synthesis will immediately result in glucocorticoid insufficiency.[16]

Critical illness may result in decreased CRH, ACTH, or cortisol synthesis through damage to the hypothalamus, pituitary gland, and/or adrenal glands. Necrosis and hemorrhage of the hypothalamus and pituitary gland have been reported in human sepsis because of prolonged hypotension or severe coagulopathy.[17] Thrombosis and hemorrhage of the adrenal glands have also been proposed as a cause of CIRCI in human critically ill patients.[3,11] Animal studies have shown that septic shock can produce extensive pathology of the adrenal glands.[11,18] For example, hemorrhagic necrosis, massive hematomas, microthrombi, and platelet aggregation have been documented in the adrenal cortices of study animals with septic shock.[18] Bilateral adrenal hemorrhage has been found in up to 30% of human critically ill patients who do not survive septic shock.[19] Occasionally, CIRCI can result from pituitary infarction secondary to traumatic injury or thrombosis.[3,11,20]

Suppression of CRH synthesis during sepsis may result from neuronal apoptosis, which may be triggered by elevation in substance P or inducible nitric oxide synthase in the hypothalamus.[21,22] Circulating proinflammatory mediators such as TNF-α may block CRH-induced ACTH release.[23] Similarly, local expression of TNF-α and IL-1β may interfere with CRH and ACTH syntheses.[22] TNF-α may also inhibit ACTH-induced cortisol release.[24] In addition, corticostatins, such as α-defensins, compete with ACTH at their membrane-binding receptor sites and exert an inhibitory effect on adrenal cells.[25]

Numerous drugs that are commonly used in critically ill patients are known to affect the HPA axis and may ultimately decrease cortisol synthesis. It is suspected that these drugs contribute, at least in part, to CIRCI.[16] Benzodiazepine administration results in a dose-dependent decrease in serum cortisol concentrations.[26] Opioid administration also results in decreased cortisol concentrations.[27] Anesthesia in humans with high-dose diazepam and fentanyl inhibits the early increase in ACTH and cortisol that occurs in response to surgery, suggesting that these drugs act at the level of the hypothalamus.[16,28] Discontinuing or reducing the dose of these drugs may result in clinical improvement in patients with CIRCI.[29]

Cortisol is synthesized via a series of cytochrome-mediated enzymatic reactions from cholesterol. Statins are thought to decrease the available substrate for cortisol synthesis, thereby decreasing overall cortisol secretion. A recent study in humans with diabetes demonstrated a dose-dependent effect of statins on cortisol production.[30]

Several drugs are known to block enzymatic steps such as the partial or complete inhibition of 11β-hydroxylase by etomidate, ketoconazole, or high-dose fluconazole.[16,31] Etomidate inhibits steroidogenesis by blocking mitochondrial cytochrome P450 enzymes, and this effect may persist as long as 24 hours after a single dose of etomidate in human critically ill patients.[32] A study of canine surgical patients demonstrated that adrenocortical function was depressed for up to 6 hours after a single intravenous (IV) bolus injection of etomidate for inducing anesthesia.[33] A similar study demonstrated that response to ACTH stimulation was also depressed 2 hours after a single IV bolus injection of etomidate in canine surgical patients.[34] In addition, a feline study found profound cortisol suppression up to 5.5 hours after the administration of a single IV bolus injection of etomidate to induce anesthesia.[35] Azole antifungals have long been associated with adrenal suppression via their ability to inhibit cytochrome P450-dependent enzymes involved in steroidogenesis. These agents differ in their inhibitory potency and selectivity for the cytochrome P450 system. Adrenal suppression is best documented with ketoconazole, and although in vitro data suggest that adrenal suppression is unlikely with triazole antifungals (eg, fluconazole and itraconazole), several human case reports have documented reversible adrenal suppression in association with these agents.[36,37] Dexmedetomidine, a highly selective and potent alpha-2 agonist, is increasingly being used for perioperative sedation and analgesia. It is an imidazole compound, and in vitro and in vivo canine studies have shown that dexmedetomidine inhibits cortisol synthesis.[38]

P-glycoprotein appears to be an important component of the HPA axis in dogs.[39] P-glycoprotein restricts the entry of cortisol into the brain, limiting cortisol's feedback inhibition of CRH and ACTH. In ABCB1 (formerly referred to as MDR1) mutant dogs, P-glycoprotein is not present, allowing greater concentrations of cortisol to be present within the brain, resulting in greater feedback inhibition of the HPA axis and, ultimately, inhibition of sufficient cortisol secretion. Plasma basal and ACTH-stimulated cortisol concentrations are significantly lower in ABCB1 mutant dogs compared with ABCB1 wild-type dogs, indicating that the HPA axis is suppressed in ABCB1 mutant dogs compared with ABCB1 wild-type dogs.[39] This may lead to an inability to appropriately respond to critical illness and stress in dogs that harbor the ABCB1 mutation. The ABCB1 mutation has been identified in herding breed dogs, such as Collies, Shetland Sheepdogs, Old English Sheepdogs, and Australian Shepherds. It has also been found at a higher frequency in sight hounds, such as Long-haired Whippets and Silken Windhounds, and also in McNabs.[40]

Reduced Access of Glucocorticoids to the Target Tissues and Cells

CBG is crucial in transporting cortisol to tissues and cells. Reductions in circulating CBG result in decreased access of cortisol to the sites of inflammation and to immune cells.[16] In human critically ill patients, CBG and albumin concentrations can decrease by approximately 50% because of catabolism at inflammatory sites and inhibition of hepatic synthesis via cytokine induction.[14] In addition, the presence of elastase is essential for cortisol cleavage and release from CBG.[16] Therefore, drugs that inhibit elastase (eg, protease inhibitors such as amprenavir, lopinavir, nelfinavir, and ritonavir) could prevent cortisol release from CBG and subsequent access to the tissue.[16] At present, protease inhibitors are not commonly used as therapeutic agents in veterinary medicine. Tissue concentrations of cortisol are also regulated by enzymatic conversion of cortisol to its inactive form, cortisone, by 11β-hydroxysteroid dehydrogenase type 2. Cytokines such as IL-2, IL-4, and IL-13 have been shown to stimulate 11β-hydroxysteroid dehydrogenase type 2 activity, converting cortisol to cortisone.[41] This inappropriate response to inflammation could be detrimental to the patient's response to illness or stress if cortisol is preferentially being converted to an inactive form. In addition, there may be a cytokine-mediated response, resulting in a decrease in the number and activity of the glucocorticoid receptors. Mechanisms may include inhibition of glucocorticoid receptor translocation from cytoplasm to nucleus and reduction in glucocorticoid receptor–mediated gene transcription.[42] This decrease would reduce the ability of cells to respond to cortisol. These different mechanisms responsible for reducing glucocorticoid access to tissues and cells could account for a decreased activity of glucocorticoids, although serum cortisol concentrations appear appropriate.[16]

INCIDENCE OF CIRCI

The incidence of CIRCI in human critically ill patients is variable and depends on the underlying disease and severity of the illness. The overall incidence of CIRCI in high-risk critically ill patients (eg, those with hypotension, shock, and sepsis) approximates 30% to 45%. The incidence increases with severity of illness (sepsis >elective surgery >ward admits), with most studies of critically ill patients reporting incidences between 25% and 40%. The incidence also depends on the specific tests and criteria used to diagnose CIRCI.[8,11,43] The ACTH stimulation test is usually used to assess adrenocortical function, but this is an area of great controversy in the human critical care arena. At present, there is no consensus for appropriately interpreting the results of ACTH stimulation testing in seriously ill patients, as accepted reference ranges are derived from healthy populations. Lack of an appropriately high basal cortisol concentration or a negligible response to ACTH may actually represent CIRCI or an insufficient response to stress in a critically ill patient.[8]

At present, little information is available regarding the incidence of CIRCI in critically ill animals with severe disease or injury. To date, there have only been a few studies that have investigated pituitary-adrenal function in populations of critically ill dogs and cats. Earlier studies evaluating pituitary-adrenal function in critically ill dogs[44] and in dogs with severe illness attributable to non–adrenal gland disease[45] did not identify any dogs with adrenal insufficiency. Prittie and colleagues[44] measured serial plasma concentrations of basal cortisol and ACTH-stimulated cortisol in 20 critically ill dogs within 24 hours of admission to an intensive care unit (ICU) and daily until death, euthanasia, or discharge from the ICU. ACTH stimulation testing was performed by IV administration of 250 µg of cosyntropin/dog. The study population was heterogeneous and consisted of animals with a variety of acute and chronic illnesses. Only 40% of the dogs enrolled in this study were acutely ill. The investigators found that basal and ACTH-stimulated cortisol concentrations were within or above the reference range in all the blood samples collected, concluding that none of the critically ill dogs developed adrenal insufficiency during hospitalization in the ICU. Delta cortisol concentrations (ACTH-stimulated cortisol concentration minus basal cortisol concentration) were not evaluated in this study. Kaplan and colleagues[45] also investigated a general population of severely ill dogs with a wide array of diseases. Most dogs studied had chronic diseases with the duration of morbidity ranging from 1 week to 1 year (mean, 5.8 ± 1.4 weeks). ACTH stimulation testing was performed by IV administration of 10 µg/kg of cosyntropin. Investigators did not identify any dogs with basal or ACTH-stimulated cortisol concentrations below the reference range. In this study, delta cortisol concentrations were not assessed.

In a more recent study, Burkitt and colleagues[46] assessed pituitary-adrenal function in 33 septic dogs admitted to an ICU. Dogs were included in the study if they had a known or suspected infectious disease and demonstrated signs consistent with systemic inflammatory response syndrome. Systemic inflammatory response syndrome was considered present if dogs demonstrated at least 2 of the following abnormalities at the time of inclusion in the study: rectal temperature more than 103.0°F or less than 100°F, heart rate more than 120 beats/min, nonpanting respiratory rate more than 40 breaths/min or Pco_2 (arterial or venous) less than 32 mm Hg, and total white blood cell count more than 16,000/µL, less than 6000/µL, or more than 3% bands. Serum cortisol and plasma endogenous ACTH concentrations were measured before and serum cortisol concentration was measured 1 hour after intramuscular administration of 250 µg of cosyntropin/dog. Basal plasma endogenous ACTH and ACTH-stimulated serum cortisol concentrations below the reference range were detected, and delta cortisol concentrations of 3 µg/dL (83 nmol/L) or less were associated with systemic hypotension and a decrease in survival. The mortality rate in dogs with delta cortisol concentrations of 3 µg/dL (83 nmol/L) or less was 4.1 times higher than that of dogs with delta cortisol concentrations more than 3 µg/dL (83 nmol/L).

The study identified CIRCI in 48% of the septic dogs enrolled in the study; however, the investigators never clearly defined the criteria used to diagnose CIRCI in their study population. Their definition was likely based on the delta cortisol concentration.

In a multicenter study[47] performed to evaluate pituitary-adrenal function in 31 acutely ill dogs with sepsis, severe trauma, or gastric dilatation-volvulus, biochemical abnormalities of the HPA axis indicating adrenal or pituitary gland insufficiency were found to be common. Serum cortisol and plasma endogenous ACTH concentrations were measured before and serum cortisol concentration was measured 1 hour after IV administration of 5 μg/kg of cosyntropin (up to a maximum of 250 μg/dog). Basal and ACTH-stimulated serum cortisol concentrations and basal plasma endogenous ACTH concentrations were assayed for each dog within 24 hours of admission to the ICU. Delta cortisol concentrations were also assessed for each patient. Overall, 55% of the critically ill dogs had at least 1 biochemical abnormality suggesting adrenal or pituitary gland insufficiency (ACTH-stimulated cortisol concentration less than the reference range, no response to ACTH stimulation [delta cortisol concentration ≤1 nmol/L], and plasma endogenous ACTH concentration less than the reference range). Only 1 dog had an exaggerated response to ACTH stimulation. Acutely ill dogs with delta cortisol concentrations of 3 μg/dL (83 nmol/L) or less were 5.7 times more likely to be receiving vasopressors than dogs with delta cortisol concentrations more than 3 μg/dL (83 nmol/L). In addition, dogs with delta cortisol concentrations of 3 μg/dL (83 nmol/L) or less had a slight, but not significant, increase in mortality. No differences were detected among dogs with sepsis, severe trauma, or gastric dilatation-volvulus with respect to mean basal and ACTH-stimulated serum cortisol concentrations, delta cortisol concentrations, and basal plasma endogenous ACTH concentrations.

Canine studies examining HPA axis function have also been performed in dogs with neoplasia (lymphoma and several different types of nonhematopoietic tumors),[48] babesiosis,[49,50] parvovirus,[51] and the ABCB1 genetic mutation.[39] Boozer and colleagues[48] investigated HPA function in dogs with lymphoma and with nonhematopoietic tumors (transitional cell carcinoma, hepatocellular adenoma, hepatocellular carcinoma, hemangiosarcoma, mammary carcinoma, jejunal adenocarcinoma, anal sac apocrine gland adenocarcinoma, insulinoma, osteosarcoma, and pheochromocytoma). None of the dogs had received any drugs known to affect adrenal function within 30 days before evaluation. Of the dogs with lymphoma and nonhematopoietic tumors, 5% and 13%, respectively, had basal cortisol concentrations below the reference range; 20% of the dogs with lymphoma and 13% of the dogs with nonhematopoietic tumors had ACTH-stimulated cortisol concentrations below the reference range. Endogenous ACTH concentrations were below the reference range in 10% of the dogs with lymphoma and 7% with nonhematopoietic neoplasia.[48] Delta cortisol concentrations were not assessed as part of the study, and the investigators did not distinguish between dogs that had absolute adrenal insufficiency or CIRCI in the tumor-bearing dogs that had HPA axis abnormalities.

Two studies have examined the endocrine response to canine babesiosis. The first study was designed, in part, to determine the association between the hormones of the pituitary-adrenal axis and outcome in dogs with naturally occurring Babesia canis rossi babesiosis.[49] In this study, basal cortisol and endogenous ACTH concentrations were measured; ACTH stimulation testing was not performed. The results indicated that serum cortisol and endogenous ACTH concentrations were significantly higher in dogs with babesiosis that died, compared with hospitalized dogs with babesiosis that survived and dogs with babesiosis that were treated as outpatients. Mortality was significantly associated with high serum cortisol and high endogenous ACTH concentrations in the dogs suffering from babesiosis. In the second study investigating endocrine response to babesiosis,[50] basal serum cortisol and plasma endogenous ACTH concentrations were measured, ACTH stimulation testing was performed, and delta cortisol concentrations and cortisol-to-ACTH ratios (which is thought by some to assess the whole pituitary-adrenal axis) were calculated. Basal serum cortisol concentrations, but not ACTH-stimulated serum cortisol concentrations, were significantly higher in the dogs with babesiosis compared with the control dogs. Basal and ACTH-stimulated serum cortisol concentrations were significantly higher in the dogs that died, compared with hospitalized dogs that survived and dogs treated as outpatients. Basal plasma endogenous ACTH concentrations were not significantly different between the 3 babesiosis groups (hospitalized dogs that died, hospitalized dogs that survived, and dogs treated as outpatients). Dogs with delta cortisol concentrations less than 83 nmol/L had significantly higher cortisol-to-ACTH ratios compared with dogs with delta cortisol concentrations more than 83 nmol/L. The investigators concluded that the findings of increased basal and ACTH-stimulated cortisol concentrations and increased cortisol-to-ACTH ratios confirmed the absence of CIRCI and demonstrated upregulation of the HPA axis in this population of dogs with acute canine critical illness.

In a study that examined puppies with parvovirus and endocrine response to illness,[51] daily IV ACTH stimulation tests were performed. Investigators found that on days 1 and 2, nonsurviving puppies with parvovirus had significantly lower delta cortisol concentrations than surviving puppies. However, on day 3, there was no statistical difference in delta cortisol concentrations between the nonsurvivors and survivors, mainly because of reduction in basal cortisol concentrations (and therefore increased delta cortisol concentrations) in the nonsurvivors, illustrating that the test results obtained on a single day do not necessarily reflect the findings on subsequent days.

The HPA axis has also been evaluated in dogs possessing the ABCB1 genetic mutation.[39] The investigators found that basal cortisol and ACTH-stimulated cortisol concentrations were significantly lower in ABCB1 mutant dogs compared with ABCB1 wild-type dogs. Plasma ACTH concentrations after dexamethasone administration were significantly lower in ABCB1 mutant dogs compared with ABCB1 wild-type dogs. The investigators concluded that the HPA axis in ABCB1 mutant dogs that lack P-glycoprotein is suppressed compared with that in ABCB1 wild-type dogs. In addition, this may explain some clinical observations in breeds known to harbor the genetic mutation, including Collies, Shelties, and Australian Shepherds. There is a clinical impression that many of these dogs have worse outcomes in response to stress and, at times, respond poorly to appropriate therapy. HPA axis suppression, secondary to the ABCB1 mutation, could result in a CIRCI-like state during times of severe stress and illness. However, further studies are required to determine the exact relationship between the ABCB1 genotype and CIRCI.

Studies investigating the presence of CIRCI in critically ill cats have also been performed. Prittie and colleagues[52] have investigated the effects of critical illness on adrenocortical function in a feline population. Twenty critically ill cats with different diseases were admitted to an ICU and constituted the study population. Plasma concentrations of basal cortisol and ACTH-stimulated cortisol were analyzed, and delta cortisol concentrations were calculated. Initial samples for basal cortisol concentrations were collected within 24 hours of admission. Samples for ACTH-stimulated cortisol concentrations were collected 1 hour after IV administration of 125 μg of cosyntropin/cat. ACTH stimulation tests were performed every other day for each cat until death or discharge from the hospital. Established reference ranges for 10 healthy cats were used for comparative purposes. The investigators found that critically ill cats had higher basal cortisol concentrations than the control group. ACTH-stimulated cortisol concentrations did not differ significantly between the 2 groups. Basal cortisol, ACTH-stimulated cortisol, and delta cortisol concentrations did not differ significantly between cats that survived and cats that died, or between the septic and nonseptic cats. However, critically ill cats with neoplasia had lower delta cortisol concentrations and were more likely to die than other cats in the study population. Based on these findings, the investigators postulated that critically ill cats with neoplasia may develop CIRCI.

Pituitary-adrenal function has been evaluated in cats with lymphoma.[53] In this study, cats with cytologic or histologic confirmation of lymphoma were investigated. None of the cats were thought to have invasion of their lymphoma to the adrenal glands, and none had received any drugs known to affect adrenal function within 30 days before evaluation. However, it should be noted that a limitation of this study was that ultrasonography was used to make the determination that there was no invasion of the lymphoma to the adrenal glands. All study cats had normal adrenal gland size, as assessed by ultrasonography. No histologic or cytologic analysis was performed to confirm that the adrenal glands were normal. Samples for basal serum cortisol, ACTH-stimulated serum cortisol, and plasma endogenous ACTH concentrations were collected and analyzed. ACTH-stimulated cortisol concentrations were collected 1 hour after IV administration of 125 μg of cosyntropin/cat. Of the 10 cats studied, 9 had a subnormal cortisol response to ACTH stimulation and 5 had elevated plasma endogenous ACTH concentrations. Based on these findings, the authors concluded that many of these cats had CIRCI. Basal cortisol concentrations and serum sodium-to-potassium ratios remained within the normal range in almost all cats, and none of the cats displayed any signs typical for complete adrenal crisis. The investigators speculated that the CIRCI present in some cats with untreated lymphoma may cause the dramatic clinical response to glucocorticoid supplementation before the induction of chemotherapy.

In a prospective multicenter study,[54] cats were enrolled if they had a known or suspected focus of infection combined with 2 or more of the following criteria: temperature more than 103.5°F or less than 100°F, heart rate less than 225 beats/min or less than 140 beats/min, respiratory rate more than 40 breaths/min, white blood cell count more than 19,500/μL, less than 5000/μL, more than 5% bands; or Doppler (systolic) blood pressure less than 90 mm Hg. Nineteen septic cats were included in the study, and 19 healthy cats served as controls. ACTH stimulation testing was performed using 125 μg of cosyntropin/cat intramuscularly. Cortisol and aldosterone concentrations were measured before and 30 minutes after ACTH administration. Delta cortisol and aldosterone concentrations were also assessed. Delta cortisol concentrations were significantly lower in septic cats (64 ± 69 nmol/L) compared with healthy cats (180 ± 129 nmol/L). Basal and post-ACTH median aldosterone concentrations were significantly higher in the septic cats (1881 and 2180 pmol/L) compared with the healthy cats (101 and 573 pmol/L), but delta aldosterone concentrations were not significantly different between the 2 groups. There was no significant difference in either delta cortisol or delta aldosterone concentration when survivors were compared with nonsurvivors.

CLINICAL SIGNS

Clinical signs of CIRCI can be vague and nonspecific, such as depression, weakness, fever, vomiting, diarrhea, and abdominal pain.[3,11,55,56] In addition, clinical signs that are secondary to the underlying disease process responsible for CIRCI (ie, septic shock, hepatic disease, trauma, etc) can mask the clinical features of CIRCI.[11] The most common clinical abnormality associated with CIRCI in human critically ill patients is hypotension refractory to fluid resuscitation, requiring vasopressor therapy.[3,8,11] Hyponatremia and hyperkalemia are uncommon in humans with CIRCI and, to date, have not been reported in canine or feline critically ill patients with insufficient adrenal or pituitary function.[3,46,47,52–54,57–59] Laboratory assessment of human critically ill patients with CIRCI may demonstrate eosinophilia and/or hypoglycemia, but these abnormalities are not consistently found in humans with CIRCI.[3,11,56] Eosinophilia and hypoglycemia have not been reported in veterinary critically ill patients with CIRCI.

DIAGNOSIS

CIRCI should be considered as a differential diagnosis in all critically ill patients requiring vasopressor support. Human patients with CIRCI typically have normal or elevated basal serum cortisol concentrations and a blunted response to ACTH stimulation.[10,60,61] These findings have also been documented in critically ill dogs with sepsis/septic shock, trauma, and gastric dilatation-volvulus and in critically ill cats with sepsis/septic shock, trauma, and neoplasia.[46,47,53,62,63] At present, there is no consensus regarding the identification of patients with CIRCI in human or veterinary medicine, and normal reference ranges do not exist for basal and ACTH-stimulated cortisol concentrations in critically ill dogs and cats.

A variety of tests have been advocated, including random basal cortisol concentration, ACTH-stimulated cortisol concentration, delta cortisol concentration (the difference when subtracting basal from ACTH-stimulated cortisol concentration), the cortisol-to-endogenous ACTH ratio, and combinations of these methods. The optimal way to identify critically ill veterinary patients with CIRCI has yet to be determined. Evaluation of adrenal function in veterinary patients typically involves administration of an ACTH stimulation test. The most commonly used protocol for ACTH stimulation testing in dogs involves the IV administration of 5 μg cosyntropin/kg up to a maximum of 250 μg. In cats, IV administration of 125 μg of cosyntropin/cat is commonly used. Serum or plasma is then obtained for cortisol analysis before and 60 minutes after ACTH administration for both dogs and cats. The standard doses of cosyntropin (5 μg/kg in dogs and 125 μg/cat) currently used in ACTH stimulation testing are greater than that necessary to produce maximal adrenocortical stimulation in healthy small animals.[64,65] Doses as low as 0.5 μg/kg in dogs[64] and 5 μg/kg in cats[65] have been shown to induce maximal cortisol secretion by the adrenal glands. The use of higher doses is considered supraphysiologic and may hinder the identification of dogs and cats with CIRCI. Low-dose (0.5 μg/kg IV) ACTH stimulation testing has been compared with standard-dose (5 μg/kg IV) ACTH stimulation testing in a group of critically ill dogs.[66] In this study, every critically ill dog that was identified to have insufficient adrenal function (ie, ACTH-stimulated serum cortisol concentration below the reference range or less than 5% greater than the basal cortisol concentration) by the standard-dose ACTH stimulation test was also identified by the low-dose test. Additional dogs with adrenal insufficiency were identified by the low-dose ACTH stimulation test and not by the standard-dose test. ACTH administered at a dose of 0.5 μg/kg IV appears to be at least as accurate in determining adrenal function in critically ill dogs as the IV administration of ACTH at 5 μg/kg. The low-dose ACTH stimulation test may even be a more sensitive diagnostic test in detecting patients with insufficient adrenal gland function than the standard-dose test.

Assays that measure cortisol concentration typically measure total hormone concentration (ie, serum free cortisol concentration plus a protein-bound fraction).

However, the serum free cortisol fraction is thought to be responsible for the physiologic function of the hormone.[67–71] Therefore, serum free cortisol concentrations may be a more precise predictor of adrenal gland function. The relationship between free and total cortisol varies with serum protein concentration.[68,69] In human critically ill patients, cortisol-binding globulin and albumin concentrations can decrease by approximately 50% because of catabolism at the inflammatory sites and inhibition of hepatic synthesis via cytokine induction.[69] Therefore, serum total cortisol concentration may be falsely low in hypoproteinemic patients, resulting in overestimation of CIRCI.[68] Serum free cortisol concentration is less likely to be altered in states of hypoproteinemia. Consequently, serum total cortisol concentrations may not accurately represent the biologic activity of serum free cortisol during critical illness. Several human studies suggest that serum free cortisol concentrations are a more accurate measure of circulating corticosteroid activity than total cortisol concentrations.[67–70] At this time, abundant canine and feline studies are lacking and the ability to measure serum free cortisol concentration is not widely available. However, serum free and total cortisol concentrations have been compared in a group of 35 critically ill dogs having 1 of the following diseases: sepsis, severe trauma, or gastric dilatation-volvulus.[66] Fewer critically ill dogs with adrenal insufficiency (ie, an ACTH-stimulated serum cortisol concentration below the reference range or less than 5% greater than the basal cortisol concentration) were identified by serum free cortisol concentration than by serum total cortisol concentration. However, basal and ACTH-stimulated serum total cortisol concentrations were not lower in the hypoproteinemic dogs compared with the normoproteinemic dogs. The significance of this is unknown and warrants further investigation in veterinary patients.

The delta cortisol concentration has been advocated as a method to identify critically ill patients with CIRCI in both human and veterinary medicine.[46,72,73] A study in human patients with septic shock[72] found that basal cortisol concentrations of 34 μg/dL (938 nmol/L) or less combined with delta cortisol concentrations of 9 μg/dL (250 nmol/L) or more in response to an IV 250 μg/person ACTH stimulation test were associated with a favorable prognosis. In addition, basal cortisol concentrations more than 34 μg/dL (938 nmol/L) combined with delta cortisol concentrations less than 9 μg/dL (250 nmol/L) were associated with a poor prognosis. Because this protocol was successful in predicting outcome, a delta cortisol concentration less than 9 μg/dL (250 nmol/L) is frequently used as the diagnostic criteria for CIRCI in human critically ill patients.

Veterinary studies have also assessed delta cortisol concentration as a criterion for diagnosing CIRCI in critically ill patients.[46,47] One study found that septic dogs with delta cortisol concentrations of 3 μg/dL (83 nmol/L) or less after an intramuscular 250 μg/dog ACTH stimulation test were more likely to have systemic hypotension and decreased survival.[46] In addition, another study investigating acutely ill dogs (ie, dogs with sepsis, severe trauma, or gastric volvulus-dilatation) found that dogs with delta cortisol concentrations of 3 μg/dL (83 nmol/L) or less after an IV 5 μg/kg ACTH stimulation test were more likely to require vasopressor therapy as part of their treatment plan.[47] Sensitivity of delta cortisol concentrations of 3 μg/dL (83 nmol/L) or less in the diagnosis of veterinary critically ill patients with CIRCI has yet to be determined.

Based on the current veterinary literature, there are 3 scenarios that may indicate the presence of CIRCI in critically ill dogs (especially in the presence of refractory hypotension): (1) dogs with a normal or an elevated basal cortisol concentration and an ACTH-stimulated cortisol concentration less than the normal reference range; (2) dogs with a normal or an elevated basal cortisol concentration and an ACTH-stimulated cortisol concentration that is less than 5% greater than the basal cortisol concentration (flatline response); and (3) dogs with a delta cortisol concentration of 3 µg/dL (83 nmol/L) or less. Based on a few clinical studies and case reports, CIRCI appears to occur in cats.[52–54,63] However, a consensus regarding the diagnostic criteria in cats is undetermined at this time.

TREATMENT

Human critically ill patients with CIRCI who are treated with supplemental doses of corticosteroids are more likely to be quickly weaned from vasopressor therapy and ventilatory support, and some treated populations of critically ill patients are more likely to survive than patients with CIRCI who do not receive corticosteroid supplementation.[60,73–76] The optimal dose and duration of treatment with corticosteroids in human patients with CIRCI have yet to be determined. The dosages of corticosteroids used to treat human patients with CIRCI are referred to as supplemental, physiologic, supraphysiologic, low dose, stress dose, or replacement.[3,8,60,73–75,77] Most human protocols have used dosages of 200 to 300 mg IV every 24 hours of hydrocortisone for an average person of 70 kg (2.9–4.3 mg/kg IV every 24 hours). The total daily dose is typically either given as a constant-rate infusion or quartered and given every 6 hours.[3,78,79] Hydrocortisone is one-forth as potent as prednisone and one-thirtieth as potent as dexamethasone. Therefore, this supplemental corticosteroid dosage is 0.7 to 1 mg/kg every 24 hours of prednisone equivalent or 0.1 to 0.4 mg/kg every 24 hours of dexamethasone equivalent. The hydrocortisone dose currently recommended for CIRCI in human patients is supraphysiologic (the human physiologic dose of hydrocortisone is 0.2–0.4 mg/kg every 24 hours), resulting in a serum cortisol concentration several times higher than that achieved by ACTH stimulation. This regimen of therapy was initially based on the maximum secretory rate of cortisol found in humans after a major surgery.[80]

At present, there are no consensus guidelines for the treatment of CIRCI in veterinary critically ill patients. However, it is reasonable to start volume-resuscitated vasopressor-dependent animals on corticosteroid therapy after performing an ACTH stimulation test. When the test results are available, treatment can be withdrawn in those animals that responded normally to the ACTH stimulation test. Corticosteroids can be continued in those patients that have (1) a normal or an elevated basal cortisol concentration and an ACTH-stimulated cortisol concentration less than the normal reference range, (2) a normal or an elevated basal cortisol concentration and an ACTH-stimulated cortisol concentration that is less than 5% greater than the basal cortisol concentration (flatline response), (3) a delta cortisol concentration of 3 µg/dL (83 nmol/L) or less, or (4) clinically demonstrated a significant improvement in cardiovascular status within 24 hours of starting corticosteroid therapy.

The appropriate dosage, duration, and type of corticosteroid therapy are unknown in veterinary patients with CIRCI. However, it is reasonable to give supplemental doses of corticosteroids at physiologic to supraphysiologic dosages (1–4.3 mg/kg IV every 24 hours of hydrocortisone [the total daily dose can be divided into 4 equal doses and given every 6 hours or as a constant-rate infusion], 0.25–1 mg/kg IV every 24 hours of prednisone equivalent [the total daily dose can be divided into 2 equal doses and given every 12 hours], or 0.04–0.4 mg/kg IV every 24 hours of dexamethasone equivalent). Because the HPA dysfunction in CIRCI is thought to be transient, lifelong therapy with corticosteroids is not required and is tapered after resolution of critical illness. The corticosteroid dose can be tapered by 25% each day. An ACTH stimulation test should be repeated to confirm the return of normal adrenocortical function following the resolution of critical illness and discontinuation of corticosteroid supplementation.

Evaluating adrenal function in human and veterinary critically ill patients can be challenging, and at present, there is no consensus regarding the identification of patients with CIRCI in human or veterinary medicine. Detection of abnormal responses will continue to be debated until standard diagnostic methods are developed and validated. At present, there are no guidelines for the treatment of CIRCI in veterinary critically ill patients, and the question as to whether supplemental doses of corticosteroids are beneficial for the treatment of CIRCI in these patients remains unanswered. Practitioners should rely on both biochemical and clinical assessment to optimize patient management.

REFERENCES

1. Jarek M, Legare E, McDermott M, et al. Endocrine profiles for outcome prediction from the intensive care unit. Crit Care Med 1993;21(4):543–50.
2. Elliott E, King L, Zerbe C. Thyroid hormone concentrations in critically ill canine patients. J Vet Emerg Crit Care 1995;5(1):17–23.
3. Cooper MS, Stewart PM. Corticosteroid insufficiency in acutely ill patients. N Engl J Med 2003;348(8):727–34.
4. Munck A, Guyre PM, Holbrook NJ. Physiologic functions of glucocorticoids in stress and their relation to pharmacological actions. Endocr Rev 1984;5(1):25–44.
5. Drucker D, Shandling M. Variable adrenocortical function in acute medical illness. Crit Care Med 1985;13(6):477–9.
6. Jurney T, Cockrell J, Lindberg J, et al. Spectrum of serum cortisol response to ACTH in ICU patients. Chest 1987;92(2):292–5.
7. Moran J, Chapman M, O'Fathartaigh M, et al. Hypocortisolemia and adrenocortical responsiveness at onset of septic shock. Intensive Care Med 1994;20(7): 489–95.
8. Beishuizen A, Thijs L. Relative adrenal failure in intensive care: an identifiable problem requiring treatment? Best Pract Res Clin Endocrinol Metab 2001;15(4): 513–31.
9. Soni A, Pepper GM, Wyrwinski PM, et al. Adrenal insufficiency occurring during septic shock: incidence, outcome, and relationship to peripheral cytokine levels. Am J Med 1995;98(3):266–71.
10. Sibbald W, Short A, Cohen M, et al. Variations in adrenocortical responsiveness during severe bacterial infections. Ann Surg 1977;186(1):29–33.
11. Zaloga GP, Marik P. Hypothalamic-pituitary-adrenal insufficiency. Crit Care Clin 2001;17(1):25–41.
12. Lamberts SWJ, Bruining HA, de Jong FH. Corticosteroid therapy in severe illness. N Engl J Med 1997;337(18):1285–92.
13. Pemberton PA, Stein PE, Pepys MB, et al. Hormone binding globulins undergo serpin conformational change in inflammation. Nature 1988;336(6196):257–8.
14. Hammond GL, Smith CL, Paterson NA, et al. A role for corticosteroid-binding globulin in delivery of cortisol to activated neutrophils. J Clin Endocrinol Metab 1990;71(1):34–9.
15. Franchimont D, Martens H, Hagelstein MT, et al. Tumor necrosis factor alpha decreases, and interleukin-10 increases, the sensitivity of human monocytes to dexamethasone: potential regulation of the glucocorticoid receptor. J Clin Endocrinol Metab 1999;84(8):2834–9.
16. Prigent H, Maxime V, Annane D. Science review: mechanisms of impaired adrenal function in sepsis and molecular actions of glucocorticoids. Crit Care 2004;8(4):243–52.

17. Sharshar T, Annane D, Lorin de la Grandmaison G, et al. The neuropathology of septic shock: a prospective case-control study. Brain Pathol 2004;14(1):21–33.

18. Hinshaw LB, Beller BK, Chang ACK, et al. Corticosteroid/antibiotic treatment of adrenalectomized dogs challenged with lethal *E. coli*. Circ Shock 1985;16(3):265–77.

19. Annane D, Bellissant E, Bollaert PE, et al. The hypothalamo-pituitary axis in septic shock. Br J Intens Care 1996;6:260–8.

20. Oelkers W. Adrenal insufficiency. N Engl J Med 1996;335(16):1206–12.

21. Larsen PJ, Jessop D, Patel H, et al. Substance P inhibits the release of anterior pituitary adrenocorticotrophin via a central mechanism involving corticotrophin-releasing factor-containing neurons in the hypothalamic paraventricular nucleus. J Neuroendocrinol 1993;5(1):99–105.

22. Sharshar T, Gray F, de la Grandmaison GL, et al. Apoptosis of neurons in cardio-vascular autonomic centres triggered by inducible nitric oxide synthase after death from septic shock. Lancet 2003;362(9398):1799–805.

23. Gaillard RC, Turnill D, Sappino P, et al. Tumor necrosis factor alpha inhibits the hormonal response of the pituitary gland to hypothalamic releasing factors. Endocrinology 1990;127(1):101–6.

24. Jaattela M, Ilvesmaki V, Voutilainen R, et al. Tumor necrosis factor as a potent inhibitor of adrenocorticotropin-induced cortisol production and steroidogenic P450 enzyme gene expression in cultured human fetal adrenal cells. Endocrinology 1991;128(1):623–9.

25. Tominaga T, Fukata J, Voutilainen R, et al. Effects of corticostatin-I on rat adrenal cells in vitro. J Endocrinol 1990;125(2):287–92.

26. Roy-Byrne PP, Cowley DS, Hommer D, et al. Neuroendocrine effects of diazepam in panic and generalized anxiety disorders. Biol Psychiatry 1991;30(1):73–80.

27. Benyamin R, Trescot AM, Datta S, et al. Opioid complications and side effects. Pain Physician 2008;11(2):S105–20.

28. Hall GM, Lacoumenta S, Hart GR, et al. Site of action of fentanyl in inhibiting the pituitary-adrenal response to surgery in man. Br J Anaesth 1990;65(2):251–3.

29. Oltmanns KM, Fehm HL, Peters A. Chronic fentanyl application induces adreno-cortical insufficiency. J Intern Med 2005;257(5):478–80.

30. Kanat M, Serin E, Tunckale A, et al. A multi-center, open label, crossover de-signed prospective study evaluating the effects of lipid lowering treatment on steroid synthesis in patients with type 2 diabetes (MODEST Study). J Endocrinol Invest 2009;32(10):852–6.

31. Thomas Z, Bandali F, McCowen K, et al. Drug-induced endocrine disorders in the intensive care unit. Crit Care Med 2010;38(6):S219–30.

32. Absalom A, Pledger D, Kong A. Adrenocortical function in critically ill patients 24 h after a single dose of etomidate. Anaesthesia 1999;54(9):861–7.

33. Dodam JR, Kruse-Elloitt KT, Aucoin DP, et al. Duration of etomidate-induced adrenocortical suppression during surgery in dogs. Am J Vet Res 1990;51(5):786–8.

34. Kruse-Elliott KT, Swanson CR, Aucoin DP. Effects of etomidate on adrenocortical function in canine surgical patients. Am J Vet Res 1987;48(7):1098–100.

35. Moon PF. Cortisol suppression in cats after induction of anesthesia with etomi-date, compared with ketamine-diazepam combination. Am J Vet Res 1997;58(8):868–71.

36. Lionakis MS, Samonis G, Kontoyiannis DP. Endocrine and metabolic manifesta-tions of invasive fungal infections and systemic antifungal treatment. Mayo Clin Proc 2008;83(9):1046–60.

37. Albert SG, DeLeon MJ, Silverberg AB. Possible association between high-dose fluconazole and adrenal insufficiency in critically ill patients. Crit Care Med 2001;29(3):668–70.

38. Maze M, Virtanen R, Daunt D, et al. Effects of dexmedetomidine, a novel imidazole sedative-anesthetic agent, on adrenal steroidgenesis: in vivo and in vitro studies. Anesth Analg 1991;73(2):204–8.

39. Mealey KL, Gay JM, Martin LG, et al. Comparison of the hypothalamic-pituitary-adrenal axis in MDR1-1Δ and MDR1 wildtype dogs. J Vet Emerg Crit Care 2007; 17(1):61–6.

40. Mealey KL, Meurs KM. Breed distribution of the ABCB1-1Δ (multidrug sensitivity) polymorphism among dogs undergoing ABCB1 genotyping. J Am Vet Med Assoc 2008;233(6):921–4.

41. Rook G, Baker R, Walker B, et al. Local regulation of glucocorticoid activity in sites of inflammation. Insights from the study of tuberculosis. Ann N Y Acad Sci 2000;917(1):913–22.

42. Pariante CM, Pearce BD, Pisell TL, et al. The proinflammatory cytokine, interleukin-1alpha, reduces glucocorticoid receptor translocation and function. Endocrinology 1999;140(9):4359–66.

43. Marik PE, Zaloga GP. Adrenal insufficiency during septic shock. Crit Care Med 2003;31(1):141–5.

44. Prittie JE, Barton LJ, Peterson ME, et al. Pituitary ACTH and adrenocortical secretion in critically ill dogs. J Am Vet Med Assoc 2002;220(5):615–9.

45. Kaplan AJ, Peterson ME, Kemppainen RJ. Effects of disease on the results of diagnostic tests for use in detecting hyperadrenocorticism in dogs. J Am Vet Med Assoc 1995;207(4):445–51.

46. Burkitt JM, Haskins SC, Nelson RW, et al. Relative adrenal insufficiency in dogs with sepsis. J Vet Intern Med 2007;21(2):226–31.

47. Martin LG, Groman RP, Fletcher DJ, et al. Pituitary-adrenal function in dogs with acute critical illness. J Am Vet Med Assoc 2008;233(1):87–95.

48. Boozer AL, Behrend EN, Kemppainen RJ, et al. Pituitary-adrenal axis function in dogs with neoplasia. Vet Comp Oncol 2005;3(4):194–202.

49. Schoeman JP, Ree P, Herrtage ME. Endocrine predictors of mortality in canine babesiosis caused by *Babesia canis rossi*. Vet Parasitol 2007;148(2):75–82.

50. Schoeman JP, Herrtage ME. Adrenal response to the low dose ACTH stimulation test and the cortisol-to-adrenocorticotrophic hormone ratio in canine babesiosis. Vet Parasitol 2008;154(3):205–13.

51. Schoeman JP. Endocrine changes during the progression of critical illness. In: Proceedings of the 27th American College of Veterinary Internal Medicine Forum and Canadian Veterinary Medical Association Convention. Montreal (Canada); 2009. p. 405–7.

52. Prittie JE, Barton LJ, Peterson ME, et al. Hypothalmo-pituitary-adrenal (HPA) axis function in critically ill cats [abstract 17]. In: Proceedings of the 9th International Veterinary Emergency and Critical Care Symposium. New Orleans (LA); 2003. p. 771.

53. Farrelly J, Hohenhaus AE, Peterson ME, et al. Evaluation of pituitary-adrenal function in cats with lymphoma. In: Proceedings of the 19th Annual Veterinary Cancer Society Conference. Wood's Hole (MA); 1999. p. 33 [abstract: 33].

54. Costello MF, Fletcher DJ, Silverstein DC, et al. Adrenal insufficiency in feline sepsis [abstract 6]. In: Proceedings of the American College of Veterinary Emergency and Critical Care Postgraduate Course 2006: Sepsis in Veterinary Medicine. San Francisco (CA); 2006. p. 41.

55. Sakharova OV, Inzucchi SE. Endocrine assessment during critical illness. Crit Care Clin 2007;23(3):467–90.

56. Maxime V, Lesur O, Annane D. Adrenal insufficiency in septic shock. Clin Chest Med 2009;30(1):17–27.

57. Ho HC, Chapital AD, Yu M. Hypothyroidism and adrenal insufficiency in sepsis and hemorrhagic shock. Arch Surg 2004;139(11):1199–203.

58. Beishuizen A, Vermes I, Hylkema BS, et al. Relative eosinophilia and functional adrenal insufficiency in critically ill patients. Lancet 1999;353(9165):1675–6.

59. Connery LE, Coursin DB. Assessment and therapy of selected endocrine disorders. Anesthesiol Clin North Am 2004;22(1):93–123.

60. Bollaert PE, Charpentier C, Levy B, et al. Reversal of late septic shock with supraphysiologic doses of hydrocortisone. Crit Care Med 1998;26(4):645–50.

61. Rivers EP, Gaspari M, Saad GA, et al. Adrenal insufficiency in high-risk surgical ICU patients. Chest 2001;119(3):889–96.

62. Peyton JL, Burkitt JM. Critical illness-related corticosteroid insufficiency in a dog with septic shock. J Vet Emerg Crit Care 2009;19(3):262–8.

63. Durkan S, de Laforcade A, Rozanski E, et al. Suspected relative adrenal insufficiency in a critically ill cat. J Vet Emerg Crit Care 2007;17(2):197–201.

64. Martin LG, Behrend EB, Mealey KL, et al. Effect of low doses of cosyntropin on serum cortisol concentrations in clinically normal dogs. Am J Vet Res 2007; 68(5):555–60.

65. Martin LG, DeClue AE, Behrend EN, et al. Effect of low doses of cosyntropin on cortisol concentrations in clinically healthy cats. J Vet Intern Med 2009; 23(3):755.

66. Martin LG, Behrend EN, Holowaychuk MK, et al. Comparison of low-dose and standard-dose ACTH stimulation tests in critically ill dogs by assessment of serum total and free cortisol concentrations. J Vet Intern Med 2010;24(3):685–6.

67. Coolens J, Baelen HV, Heyns W. Clinical use of unbound plasma cortisol as calculated from total cortisol and corticosteroid binding globulin. J Steroid Biochem 1987;26(2):197–202.

68. Hamranian AH, Oseni TS, Arafah BM. Measurements of serum free cortisol in critically ill patients. N Engl J Med 2004;350(16):1629–38.

69. Torpy DJ, Ho JT. Value of free cortisol measurement in systemic infection. Horm Metab Res 2007;39(6):439–44.

70. Poomthavorn P, Lertbunrian R, Preutthipan A, et al. Serum free cortisol index, free cortisol, and total cortisol in critically ill children. Intensive Care Med 2009;35(7): 1281–5.

71. Kemppainen RJ, Peterson ME, Sartin JL. Plasma free cortisol concentrations in dogs with hyperadrenocorticism. Am J Vet Res 1991;52(5):682–6.

72. Annane D, Sebille V, Troche G, et al. A 3-level prognostic classification in septic shock based on cortisol levels and cortisol response to corticotropin. JAMA 2000; 283(8):1038–45.

73. Annane D, Sebille V, Charpentier C, et al. Effect of treatment with low doses of hydrocortisone and fludrocortisone on mortality in patients with septic shock. JAMA 2002;288(7):862–71.

74. Briegel J, Forst H, Haller M, et al. Stress doses of hydrocortisone reverse hyperdynamic septic shock: a prospective, randomized, double-blind, single-center study. Crit Care Med 1999;27(4):723–32.

75. Oppert M, Schindler R, Husung C, et al. Low-dose hydrocortisone improves shock reversal and reduces cytokine levels in early hyperdynamic septic shock. Crit Care Med 2005;33(11):2457–64.

76. Meduri GU, Marik PE, Chrousos GP, et al. Steroid treatment in ARDS: a critical appraisal of the ARDS network trial and the recent literature. Intensive Care Med 2008;34(1):61–9.

77. Yildiz O, Doganay M, Aygen B, et al. Physiologic-dose steroid therapy in sepsis. Crit Care 2002;6(3):251–9.

78. Prigent H, Maxime V, Annane D. Clinical review: corticotherapy in sepsis. Crit Care 2004;8(2):122–9.

79. Marik PE. Critical illness-related corticosteroid insufficiency. Chest 2009;135(1):181–93.

80. Prittie JE. Adrenal insufficiency in critical illness. In: Bonagura JB, Twedt DC, editors. Kirk's current veterinary therapy XIV. 1st edition. St Louis (MO): Saunders Elsevier; 2009. p. 228–30.

Defects in Coagulation Encountered in Small Animal Critical Care

Benjamin M. Brainard, VMD[a],*,
Andrew J. Brown, MA VetMB, MRCVS[b]

KEYWORDS

• DIC • Disseminated intravascular coagulation • Antithrombin
• Plasma • Heparin

Patients with systemic inflammatory response may develop hemostatic abnormalities, ranging from subtle and subclinical activation of coagulation to fulminant disseminated intravascular coagulation (DIC). Inflammation in these patients may be secondary to infection, trauma, pancreatitis, immune-mediated disease, or neoplasia, among other pathologies. In addition, metabolic abnormalities in the critically ill patient can result in altered hemostasis.

INFLAMMATION AND COAGULATION

Inflammation is an appropriate host response to infection or tissue damage. Activation of coagulation and intravascular thrombosis occurs in concert with inflammatory responses and acts to prevent spread of microorganisms into the systemic circulation, limit bleeding, and promote tissue repair.[1] Infectious and noninfectious insults, such as trauma, pancreatitis, immune-mediated disease, or neoplasia, can result in the systemic inflammatory response syndrome (SIRS), when the appropriate localized inflammatory response becomes a generalized reaction. Severe systemic inflammatory cytokine release, activation of leukocytes and endothelial cells, and decreased tissue oxygen delivery can eventually result in multiple organ dysfunction syndrome (MODS) and ultimately organ failure and death. As the local inflammatory response becomes a systemic response, activation of coagulation occurs, resulting in extensive formation, and subsequent fibrinolysis, of microthrombi. This widespread activation of the hemostatic system is termed disseminated intravascular coagulation. Just as SIRS has a spectrum from mild to severe inflammation, DIC can be present on a scale from

This work is unsupported by grant funding.
The authors have nothing to disclose.
[a] Department of Small Animal Medicine and Surgery, University of Georgia, 501 D.W. Brooks Drive, Athens, GA 30602, USA
[b] VetsNow Referral Hospital, 123-145 North Street, Glasgow, G3 7DA Scotland, UK
* Corresponding author.
E-mail address: brainard@uga.edu

Vet Clin Small Anim 41 (2011) 783–803
doi:10.1016/j.cvsm.2011.04.001
0195-5616/11/$ – see front matter © 2011 Elsevier Inc. All rights reserved.

vetsmall.theclinics.com

mild to severe intravascular coagulation. In its mildest form, DIC may be limited to mild intravascular thrombosis detected only by hemostatic markers. However, marked activation of coagulation and subsequent fibrinolysis can result in the development of fulminant DIC characterized by widespread microvascular thrombosis and profuse bleeding, a consumptive thrombohemorrhagic syndrome.[2] DIC has traditionally been considered a consequence of SIRS,[3–6] and, when present, is a strong predictor of the development of MODS and mortality.[7] However, there is now evidence that a bidirectional interaction between SIRS and DIC exists, which together play a significant role in the development of microvascular thrombosis, MODS, and poor prognosis in critically ill patients.[8]

INTRAVASCULAR THROMBOSIS AND COAGULOPATHY

Intravascular thrombosis is a result of activation of coagulation, inhibition of anticoagulation, and depression of fibrinolysis. A fine balance normally exists between hemostatic and fibrinolytic pathways. This delicate balance is altered by tissue injury and inflammation (both infectious and sterile). Initiation of inflammation-induced coagulation occurs by tissue factor (TF)-mediated thrombin generation.[9] Blood comes into contact with TF when blood vessel wall integrity is lost or activated endothelial cells and monocytes/macrophages express TF. Activation of platelets also results in the release of the alpha and dense granules from the platelet cytoplasm. Substances released from platelets serve to promote coagulation (TF, factors Va and VIIIa), alter vascular tone (serotonin), and activate or recruit additional platelets (ADP, P-selectin). In addition, a membrane shape change occurs and the platelets express the active form of the fibrinogen receptor (GPIIb/IIIa). Platelet activation may also contribute to TF expression, and the platelet membrane plays an important role in supporting the initiation of coagulation.[10] Following trauma, tissue injury leads to TF exposure and thrombin generation. In addition, exposed subendothelial collagen may result in platelet activation. In sepsis, initial expression of TF is mediated by proinflammatory cytokines, namely interleukin (IL)-6, tumor necrosis factor (TNF)-alpha, and IL-1 beta.[11–13] The TF-VIIa complex can also stimulate production of additional proinflammatory cytokines by upregulation of nF-kB.[14] TF is shuttled between endothelial and polymorphonuclear cells through microparticles (small, membrane-derived vesicles) released from activated mononuclear cells.[15] TF-bearing microparticles may contribute to the systemic activation of coagulation; both endothelial cells and platelets may also release microparticles into the general circulation.[16]

The endogenous anticoagulant pathways, antithrombin (AT), protein C/protein S system, and tissue-factor pathway inhibitor (TFPI) closely regulate procoagulant pathways and are all impaired during inflammation-induced coagulation. AT is the primary inhibitor of thrombin and factor Xa, and AT levels are markedly decreased during severe inflammation because of impaired synthesis, neutrophil-mediated degradation, and consumption secondary to ongoing thrombin generation.[17] Activated protein C (aPC) in concert with protein S degrades cofactors Va and VIIIa, which are essential cofactors for the intrinsic and common pathways. Similar to AT, plasma levels of zymogen protein C are decreased during severe inflammation.[18,19] Zymogen protein C is activated by thrombomodulin, which is in turn activated by thrombin. Although this balances the procoagulant response to mild inflammation, severe inflammation results in downregulation of the endothelial thrombomodulin-protein C receptor pathway[20] via activation of endothelial nF-kB.[21] Under normal conditions, the endothelial protein C receptor (EPCR) accelerates the activation of protein C (PC) and amplifies the anticoagulant and antiinflammatory effects of aPC.[22] EPCR expression is downregulated in sepsis, further reducing the effects of the protein C system. The final endogenous anticoagulant system that is affected by inflammation is TFPI, which is released from endothelial cells in response to inflammation or damage. TFPI forms a quaternary complex with factors Xa and VIIa to inhibit coagulation induced by TF.[23] Levels of TFPI in patients with sepsis are initially low, and rabbits that are depleted of TFPI are prone to intravascular coagulation, although a major multicenter trial studying the infusion of recombinant human TFPI failed to show an effect on the mortality of a group of patients with septic shock.[24]

Plasminogen activators are released into the circulation from vascular endothelial cells in response to clot formation and inflammatory mediators, such as TNF-alpha and IL-1 beta.[25] Plasminogen is converted to plasmin by specific activators, such as tissue plasminogen activator (tPA). Plasmin is then able to break down the fibrin strands that create a thrombus. The fibrinolytic action of plasminogen is balanced by a natural inhibitor, plasminogen activator inhibitor type 1 (PAI-1), which is released by endothelial cells and prevents activation of plasmin. Plasmin may be directly inactivated by circulating alpha 2-antiplasmin. In severe inflammation, there is a delayed yet sustained increase in PAI-1 that slows fibrinolysis and contributes to persistence of microvascular thrombi and thromboemboli.[26]

DIC can manifest as both diffuse intravascular thrombosis leading to organ dysfunction or a hemorrhagic phenotype characterized by excessive bleeding, which is one reason for the preference of the term "consumptive thrombohemorrhagic disorder" rather than DIC.[12] The consumptive phase of DIC uses platelets and coagulation factors (consumptive coagulopathy) to produce microthrombosis and occasionally macrothrombosis, and is associated with tPA-induced fibrino/fibrinogenolysis.[27] When platelets and hemostatic factors reach critically low levels caused by consumption, bleeding ensues.

TRAUMA AND HEMOSTASIS

Hemostatic abnormalities are common in critically ill patients following trauma, resulting in either a hypercoagulable or hypocoagulable state. Following trauma-induced tissue damage and exposure of the subendothelial layer of blood vessels, blood is exposed to TF, collagen, and von Willebrand factor (vWF). Clotting is rapidly initiated and amplified via the TF pathway following platelet activation and aggregation. The coagulation cascade is therefore an integral part of limiting hemorrhage in the trauma patient. However, the resultant hypercoagulable state after injury is thought to play a major role in the development of multiple organ dysfunction syndrome, primarily caused by microthrombosis and disruption of blood flow in end organs. MODS is the leading cause of death in people after the initial 48 hours following trauma.[28,29] MODS and DIC have also been documented in dogs secondary to trauma, and have been shown to be significantly associated with nonsurvival.[30]

Unlike DIC resulting from inflammatory conditions, the DIC-like syndrome following trauma is likely less associated with inflammation and upregulation of cellular receptors and more related to the activation of coagulation from widespread endothelial disruption. The hypovolemia and hypoperfusion that may accompany trauma also impair clearance of thrombin, allowing increased formation of thrombin-thrombomodulin complexes.[31] Subsequent activation of protein C and upregulation (decreased inhibition) of fibrinolysis can lead to a DIC-like syndrome.[31]

Subsequent to this early hypercoagulable state, blood loss, factor consumption, and fluid resuscitation may promote a systemic hypocoagulable state. The coagulopathy is initiated by consumption of factors and platelets following hemorrhage. The administration of crystalloids and colloids for resuscitation will result in a dilutional coagulopathy, and colloids will also impede the interaction of factor VIII and vWF.[32] Shock and subsequent acidosis may alter coagulation protease function and may contribute to hemorrhagic diatheses. Trauma patients are commonly hypothermic when presented to the hospital, and this can worsen a coagulopathy. A lethal triad of coagulopathy, hypothermia, and acidemia is well described.[31] Resuscitation with refrigerated blood products or room-temperature fluids may further worsen patient hypothermia, and crystalloids with a high concentration of chloride can worsen the acidosis.

DEFECTS IN HEMOSTASIS SECONDARY TO METABOLIC DISEASE

In addition to the activation and consumption of platelets and coagulation factors, animals with severe organ dysfunction may experience impaired platelet activity, which can promote bleeding and complicate therapy. Moderate to severe uremia and renal disease can result in impaired platelet secretion of ADP, serotonin, and production of thromboxane A_2 (TXA_2), as well as changes in cytoplasmic calcium dynamics.[33] Impaired expression of fibrinogen receptors and von Willebrand activity may decrease the ability of platelets to adhere to sites of injury, especially under high shear conditions.[33] Studies in dogs have documented alterations in ex vivo platelet aggregation in the presence of uremia.[34] Decreased platelet function can complicate therapies that require additional anticoagulation, such as hemodialysis. In human patients with severe acute hepatitis and encephalopathy, abnormalities of platelet function have been noted, and a study of platelet aggregation in a group of dogs with various types of liver disease showed decreased whole blood platelet aggregation responses to collagen and arachidonic acid in some dogs.[35,36] Patients with chronic liver disease may exhibit decreased platelet TXA_2 production.[36] The bone marrow of patients with various types of hematopoietic diseases may produce abnormal platelets, with incomplete or abnormal granule contents (generally referred to as acquired storage pool disease [SPD]). SPD has been described in human patients with autoimmune disease, DIC, antiplatelet antibodies, and hemangioma.[37] Although the clinical implications of some of these abnormalities in platelet function are unclear in companion animals, platelet dysfunction may compound any coagulopathy and may complicate invasive diagnostic or therapeutic procedures.

DIAGNOSIS

Although DIC frequently occurs secondary to severe sepsis, polytrauma, and other inflammatory conditions, no single clinical sign or laboratory test has been identified that possesses sufficient accuracy to confirm or reject a diagnosis.[12,38] Because it is difficult to accurately identify animals with DIC, it is important to critically assess research evaluating animals with DIC for the specific criteria used to diagnose DIC. In veterinary medicine, DIC is commonly diagnosed based upon abnormalities in at least 3 of the following hemostatic parameters: activated partial thromboplastin time (aPTT), prothrombin time PT, fibrinogen, D-dimer (DD), platelet concentration, and erythrocyte morphology, together with evidence of a predisposing condition.[39–41] Although sensitive, this is a nonspecific approach.[39–41] Because no gold standard exists in the diagnosis of DIC in either human or veterinary medicine, expert evaluation of an extended hemostatic panel has been used to increase sensitivity and specificity of diagnosis in the research setting.[40,42] The subcommittee on DIC of the Scientific and Standardization of the International Society of Thrombosis and Haemostasis has proposed a scoring system in people, based on a combination of commonly measured hemostatic parameters.[43] This scoring system was prospectively validated and was deemed sufficiently accurate to make or reject a diagnosis of DIC in intensive care patients with a clinical suspicion of DIC.[42] In addition, there was a strong correlation between DIC score and 28-day mortality. This scoring system was recently used as a template to develop a model-based scoring system for diagnosis of canine DIC.[39] The model included values for the PT, aPTT, fibrinogen, and DD concentrations, and was prospectively evaluated, with a reported sensitivity of 83.3% and specificity of 77.3% (based upon expert evaluation and diagnosis of DIC as the gold standard). In addition to those data that were included in the final model, this study evaluated platelet count, antithrombin, proteins C and S, alpha-1 antiplasmin, and plasminogen concentrations.[39]

PLATELET COUNT

Thrombocytopenia can occur secondary to increased consumption, destruction, dilution, sequestration, and decreased production. Dogs may develop thrombocytopenia secondary to sepsis, trauma, and immune-mediated hemolytic anemia (IMHA). Thrombocytopenia may also occur secondary to immune-mediated thrombocytopenia, but is beyond the scope of this review. Thrombocytopenia from DIC or other consumptive causes frequently results in a platelet count between 40 and 100 $\times$ 10^9 L^{-1}, whereas immune-mediated destruction of platelets usually results in a platelet count less than 20 $\times$ 10^9 L^{-1}. The true incidence of thrombocytopenia is unknown and in part depends on the definition. Although individual laboratories have reference intervals, it has been suggested that a threshold of 100 $\times$ 10^9 L^{-1} be termed thrombocytopenia in critically ill people[44,45] because of the high incidence and lack of significant bleeding in these patients. In critically ill people, platelet concentrations less than 100 $\times$ 10^9 L^{-1} are associated with a 10-fold increased risk of bleeding than a concentration between 100 and 150 $\times$ 10^9 L^{-1}.[46] Surgical bleeding is uncommon if platelet concentration is greater than 50 $\times$ 10^9 L^{-1} and data from human patients with cancer suggest that the risk of spontaneous bleeding does not increase until the concentration is less than 20 $\times$ 10^9 L^{-1}.[47,48] Platelet count may be estimated using many automated complete blood count machines, but it is always indicated to review a blood smear, especially in patients with severe inflammatory disease, as platelet clumping or changes in mean platelet volume can result in erroneous values. This factor is especially true in cats. When reviewing a blood smear, each platelet seen on a high power field (100X) represents approximately 15 $\times$ 10^9 L^{-1} circulating platelets.

Independent of the risk of bleeding, thrombocytopenia serves as a marker of morbidity and mortality, likely related to the severity of the underlying condition. Severity of thrombocytopenia is inversely correlated to survival in critically ill people, and sustained thrombocytopenia over 4 days is associated with a 4- to 6-fold increase in mortality.[46,49]

PROTHROMBIN AND ACTIVATED PARTIAL THROMBOPLASTIN TIME

The prothrombin time monitors the tissue factor (extrinsic) pathway and common portions of the coagulation cascade. Tissue factor and calcium are added to plasma, activating factor VII and in turn, factors X, V, and II (prothrombin). Fibrin formation from fibrinogen is the end point of the assay, measured using either optical or mechanical means, depending on the methodology. Activated partial thromboplastin time is measured in citrated plasma by adding thromboplastin or a similar source of lipoprotein, with calcium and other activators, again allowing coagulation to proceed to fibrin formation, in this case by the subsequent activation of the factors in the intrinsic pathway (factors XII, XI, IX, VIII, X, V, and II). Final fibrin formation is again monitored by optical or mechanical means. In one study, dogs with sepsis had significantly higher PT and aPTT values than controls.[50] It appears in many animals with DIC that the aPTT is the first clotting time to become prolonged, and animals with early DIC may only display a moderate prolongation of aPTT and thrombocytopenia. This combination should alert the astute clinician to monitor patients closely for progression of the syndrome.

VISCOELASTIC COAGULATION MONITORING

Viscoelastic coagulation monitors, such as thromboelastography (TEG, Haemoscope/Haemonetics, Niles, IL, USA) or Sonoclot (Sienco Inc, Arveda, CO, USA), assess the viscoelastic changes in whole blood during clot formation and provide a global assessment of hemostatic capability, because whole blood analysis integrates both cellular and plasmatic contributions to coagulation. TEG has recently been used to identify pro-thrombotic states in dogs with IMHA, neoplasia, and DIC.[40,51,52] Unlike PT and aPTT, these machines can identify both hypercoagulable and hypocoagulable states.[53] One recent study evaluating TEG in dogs with DIC demonstrated a greater fatality rate in hypocoagulable dogs than those that were hypercoagulable.[40] However, because TEG assesses whole blood, it is potentially affected by all constituent components of blood, including platelet concentration and hematocrit.[54,55] It also may be affected by contact (intrinsic) pathway activation resulting from differences in sample collection method and quality of venipuncture.[56,57] As such, these factors should be considered during interpretation of TEG and when developing reference intervals. Although the TEG is generally run at a test temperature of 37°C, the temperature of the blood sample during the rest period does not appear to result in clinically relevant differences in contact activation or TEG parameters.[58]

TEG has potential for documenting a prothrombotic state in early DIC and may therefore identify those patients that require thromboprophylaxis before the development of overt DIC. In addition, viscoelastic coagulation testing has the potential to be used to monitor patient response to therapy, allowing treatments to be tailored accordingly. The addition of specific inhibitors of platelet function or contact activation also have promise for more specific diagnosis of the components of hypercoagulable or hypocoagulable states.[59,60]

MICROPARTICLES

Microparticles (MPs) may be released from cellular sources during inflammatory conditions and can circulate systemically. Circulating MPs may be detected by the use of flow cytometry.[61,62] They have also been identified using plate adherence techniques, as well as electron microscopy.[63] Because the MPs may be of varied cellular origin (platelet, endothelial cell, monocyte), it is important, in addition to evaluating these particles for expression of markers, such as CD62P (P-selectin) and TF, to include specific markers to determine the cellular origin (eg, CD41/61 for platelet MPs and CD104 for endothelial MPs).[62] Although elevated levels of circulating MPs have been identified in human patients with trauma, neoplasia, and DIC,[64,65] the prognostic significance of this elevation is not yet clear; in some cases, elevations of MPs may indicate an appropriate response to inflammation and the potential for successful resolution of the disease.[66]

PLATELET FUNCTION ASSAYS

Platelet function defects can be difficult to evaluate in the context of some whole blood coagulation testing (eg, TEG), and may require more specific diagnostics.[67] Optical aggregometry (OA) uses a spectrophotometric technique to evaluate platelets in platelet rich plasma (PRP) for responses to various agonists and is considered the gold standard for assessment of platelet function.[68] Whole blood (impedance) aggregometry (WBA) uses an electrical probe and measures the resistance caused by platelets as they adhere to the probe after exposure to agonists, the impedance of the circuit being directly related to the degree of aggregation.[69] WBA is convenient and requires a smaller blood volume than OA, but may not be as accurate. With platelet counts less than 100 to 150 $\times$ 10^9 L^{-1}, however, the accuracy of both techniques is decreased; ideal analyses use PRP platelet counts around 300 $\times$ 10^9 L^{-1}. The platelet function analyzer (PFA-100 [Siemens Healthcare Diagnostics, Deerfield, IL, USA]) is a system that aspirates citrated whole blood through a small aperture primed with agonists for platelet aggregation (eg, collagen and ADP). The machine measures the time (up to 300 seconds) that it takes for a platelet plug to occlude the aperture (closure time).[70] The PFA-100 has been validated for use in small animal patients, and can be useful for diagnosing disorders of primary hemostasis, such as von Willebrand disease.[71,72] The accuracy of this machine is also decreased in patients with low platelet counts.[73] Other machines designed to evaluate platelet function (eg, the Impact system [Matis Medical, Beersel, Belgium]) are pending further assessment for utility in analysis of platelet function in veterinary patients. Activated platelets have been identified in many species using flow cytometry,[74–76] and as this modality becomes more available to veterinarians, may add additional diagnostic information to the state of circulating platelets in patients with DIC. Flow cytometry is not affected by patients' total platelet count, but analyses may take longer in patients who are thrombocytopenic.

ANTITHROMBIN AND PROTEIN C ACTIVITY

Antithrombin and PC are typically measured by functional activity assays compared with reference plasma. As important physiologic inhibitors of hemostasis, a decreased activity indicates a prothrombotic state. Low AT and PC activity have been identified in dogs with sepsis, IMHA and DIC, and low activity has been associated with an increased mortality risk.[40,41,50,77–80] Studies in people have suggested that serial measurements of AT and PC have prognostic utility.[7,81] A preliminary study in septic dogs was consistent with this; both PC and AT activities changed significantly over time and were associated with outcome.[77]

ASSESSMENT OF FIBRINOLYSIS

Fibrin degradation products (FDP) are the breakdown products of both fibrin and fibrinogen generated by the enzymatic action of plasmin, whereas DD result only from degradation of fibrin that is part of an intact clot (ie, has been cross-linked).[82] FDP assays lack specificity and are also insensitive for identifying thromboembolic disease[83]; as such, measuring FDP concentration is not useful in critically ill patients. Studies have demonstrated an increased DD concentration in dogs with clinical diagnoses of sepsis, IMHA, DIC, and thromboembolic disease.[50,79,83,84] The greatest utility for the DD assay is likely as an adjunct test to rule out thromboembolic disease. As DD concentrations are used primarily for negative predictive value, it is important that an ultrasensitive assay be used to avoid false-negative results.

THERAPY FOR DIC

Because DIC is a multifactorial syndrome, therapy is primarily supportive and directed toward resolution of the inciting cause. Supportive therapy should restore and maintain tissue oxygen delivery, and consideration of the pathophysiology of DIC may define additional options for therapeutic intervention.

The first aspect of therapy is treatment of the primary underlying condition; this can include surgical (eg, to drain an abscess or debride tissue) or medical (eg, antibiotics to treat sepsis) approaches. The inflammation that drives DIC may continue even after appropriate therapy is initiated. Another important part of therapy is to treat shock and to maximize oxygen delivery to the tissues. Tissue hypoxia may promote additional inflammation that can worsen SIRS and lead to MODS.

Resuscitation from shock associated with trauma should include the use of both intravenous crystalloid and colloids, in addition to the transfusion of red blood cells to preserve oxygen carrying capacity. The addition of fresh frozen plasma (FFP) to this regime may help to reverse some of the early aberrations and ameliorate the developing coagulopathy.[31] This point is especially true when treating the coagulopathy associated with trauma. Crystalloid fluids low in chloride (eg, Normosol-R or lactated Ringer's solution) should be chosen to minimize the acidosis associated with iatrogenic hyperchloremia (that may result from the use of 0.9% sodium chloride). Recent studies of humans with trauma have advocated a 1:1 or 1:2 ratio of FFP to packed red blood cells (pRBC) in patients receiving massive transfusions, although the benefit of this concept for different patient populations and those not requiring massive transfusions remains to be determined.[85]

FRESH FROZEN PLASMA

Fresh frozen plasma administration is indicated in patients with coagulopathy caused by factor deficiency, especially if hemorrhage is ongoing. Patients with significant bleeding and thrombocytopenia may benefit from a transfusion of fresh whole blood or platelet-rich plasma. A recent study evaluating the administration of a single transfusion of FFP (median 16.5 mL/kg, range 4–30 mL/kg) to dogs with pancreatitis did not demonstrate a beneficial effect from the administration of FFP.[86] In this study, only 2 dogs of 77 had evidence of coagulopathy, and 17/38 met criteria for SIRS. Platelet counts were not reported, so it cannot be determined if a subset of the studied population was experiencing DIC (although given the low incidence of coagulopathy, only 2 patients might have met the criteria for DIC). The retrospective nature of this study and the small numbers merit additional prospective studies, as well as studies of patients with other inflammatory states that can lead to DIC. It is important to note the results of a 1991 study in humans with severe acute pancreatitis, however, where high-dose FFP (8 units daily for 3 days) did not result in a difference in mortality, although this regime did result in significant improvements (ie, maintenance in the normal range) in plasma antithrombin, and α2-macroglobulin.[87] The ability of this protocol to maintain levels of antiinflammatory proteins may be applicable to other inflammatory and consumptive diseases.

Few guidelines exist in the veterinary literature for dosages for FFP transfusion.[88,89] An initial dose of 6 to 10 mL/kg is indicated for correction of coagulopathy, but hemostatic parameters should be reevaluated after therapy, and additional FFP administered if necessary. In a 3-month survey of FFP transfusions in a veterinary teaching hospital , canine patients received an average FFP dose of 9 mL/kg (ranging from 2–30 mL/kg).[90] These dogs received FFP for indications ranging from coagulopathy to replacement of plasma proteins (eg, α-macroglobulin, albumin). Although 50% of the dogs in this study received a single FFP transfusion, 46% received a FFP transfusion either twice or 3 times daily. Patient outcomes were not reported in this study. A more recent article evaluating FFP transfusion in dogs noted median transfusion volumes of 15 to 18 mL/kg.[91] This article demonstrated a significant shortening in patient PT and aPTT times in patients who were coagulopathic following plasma transfusion, although it was not able to determine whether these patients had evidence of hemorrhage or just prolonged clotting times. In a small cohort of cats (n = 46) with DIC, therapy included transfusion of a single unit (volume unspecified) of FFP in 21 cats (46%). Survival statistics were not different between cats who received FFP and those who did not.[92]

In patients with an ongoing consumptive coagulopathy, frequent redosing of FFP may help to replace coagulation factors and anticoagulant proteins. Some authors have advocated anticoagulation before FFP administration in human patients with DIC, although the implications for veterinary medicine are unclear.[93] In veterinary patients with severe inflammatory conditions and DIC, some clinicians advocate a dosing regimen of 10 mL/kg of FFP up to 3 times daily, if clinical and laboratory signs warrant. Extrapolation from human data indicates that this large amount of FFP may not be necessary, and suggests that FFP should be used only when clinically indicated by coagulopathy accompanied by hemorrhage (this is especially true in patients with sepsis). A retrospective human study has questioned even the utility of this practice, noting that patients who received FFP transfusion had a significantly higher incidence of acute lung injury, although other outcome measures were not different between groups.[94] Prospective studies of FFP use specifically in veterinary patients with inflammatory disease are indicated to better determine appropriate dosing regimens for these patients.

Although plasma or other blood product transfusions may benefit veterinary patients with DIC, the complications associated with plasma transfusions should be kept in mind. Although transfusion reactions are not frequently reported in recent veterinary studies,[86,90] all transfusions must be monitored closely. It seems logical that type-specific FFP should be administered when available, although this has not been specifically studied. Transfusion reactions can be mild, such as pruritus, facial swelling, or rash,[95] or more severe, such as fever,[96] anaphylaxis, or death. In other studies, the transfusion of perioperative blood products (FFP and pRBC) occurred more frequently in animals that developed postoperative pulmonary complications.[97] This finding raises the possibility of transfusion-related acute lung injury (TRALI), which is an acute respiratory distress syndrome (ARDS)-like event that occurs during or within 6 hours of a transfusion.[98] TRALI in humans has been associated with transfusion of both pRBCs and FFP, but has not been definitively described in the veterinary literature to date.

ANTITHROMBIN

Experimental models have suggested that the administration of antithrombin concentrate may attenuate the clinical course of DIC. AT, in combination with endogenous or exogenous heparinlike substances, promotes anticoagulation by inactivation of (primarily) factors IIa and Xa. Because thrombin (IIa) is a potent stimulus for additional coagulation, inactivation may help quell additional clot formation. In addition, AT is a potent antiinflammatory molecule, contributing to endothelial cell prostacyclin production,[99] as well as decreasing margination and leukocyte-endothelial cell interaction.[100] Prostacyclin production also inhibits platelet activation, resulting in less release of procoagulant and proinflammatory (eg, IL-1) factors.[99]

Dogs with inflammatory states and DIC have decreased AT activities, which may continue to decrease with continued inflammation and activation of coagulation.[40,77,101,102] Extensive studies have not been performed in cats with inflammatory disease,[103–105] and AT levels in cats with cardiomyopathy were in the normal range in one study and increased in another.[106,107] Despite the fact that low AT levels are associated with a poor prognosis in both dogs[40] and humans[108] with DIC, a large human study failed to show a survival benefit of AT administration, except in a subgroup that did not receive concomitant heparin.[109] In fact, the use of heparin appears to negate the benefits of AT administration and may result in an increase in bleeding complications.[110] Subsequent studies evaluating the use of AT concentrate in patients with DIC caused by sepsis or burns, while avoiding concomitant heparin therapy, have been more promising.[111,112] The binding of AT to exogenous heparin likely inhibits AT binding to endothelial cell glycosaminoglycans,[113,114] resulting in a mitigation of the antiinflammatory effects of AT.[115]

There are no current recommendations on the use of AT concentrate in small animal patients. In humans, AT concentrate is dosed to elevate AT levels to 120%.[116] Doses are calculated based on an activity elevation of 1.4% per U/kg of AT. Human FFP contains about 1 unit of AT activity per milliliter, so 10 mL/kg of FFP would be expected to provide an elevation of 14% in AT activity.[116] One study in dogs with IMHA evaluated the change in AT activity after transfusion of a single 10 mL/kg dose of FFP. In this study, there were no significant changes in AT activity after this transfusion. There was also a variable AT activity in the transfused plasma, ranging from 55% to 96%.[117] These dogs were also receiving unfractionated heparin. Similar results on AT levels were found after transfusion of 15 mL/kg of FFP in dogs with IMHA.[118] A single study that evaluated the use of human AT concentrate (administered over 90 minutes at a dose of 1 U/mL of calculated circulating canine plasma; presumably 50–60 U/kg) in dogs with experimental DIC showed less glomerular fibrin deposition and a blunted rise in FDPs compared with control dogs.[119] Experimental studies using feline AT concentrate in cats showed a decrease in thrombin-induced neutrophil rolling after ischemia and reperfusion injury, but not during lipopolysaccharide challenge.[100,120] Because human and canine and feline AT are different, the possibility exists that infusion of human AT concentrate into veterinary species could result in the formation of antihuman AT antibodies or in hypersensitivity reactions.

ACTIVATED PROTEIN C

Human studies have evaluated the administration of activated protein C to patients with severe sepsis. Under normal circumstances, thrombin bound to thrombomodulin activates PC, which, with its cofactor protein S, acts to inactivate factors Va and VIIIa. When infused intravenously (IV), aPC binds thrombomodulin and acts as a potent anticoagulant protein. Activation of the endothelial protein C receptor modulates cytokine release by interfering with NF-κB translocation, resulting in a decreased expression of cytokines by endothelial cells and interference with thrombin binding to PAR-1 receptors.[99] aPC also has a binding site on monocytes and may decrease production of proinflammatory mediators.[121] A landmark human study (PROWESS) published in 2001 showed promise that aPC could reduce mortality and organ dysfunction in patients suffering from severe sepsis.[122,123] Of note, the subgroup of patients with DIC in this study experienced a greater relative benefit from the infusion of aPC.[124]

Despite the findings of the PROWESS trial, the use of aPC in human patients with severe sepsis and DIC remains controversial. Subsequent studies and meta-analyses, specifically in patients with sepsis, have failed to provide compelling evidence for its use.[125] There is only one published study of the use of aPC in dogs, which infused 1 and 2 mg/kg/h of aPC IV for 2 hours and demonstrated a dose-dependent prolongation of aPTT (2.0- and 3.7-fold prolongation, respectively) without significant effect on platelet function or thrombin clot time.[126] These effects were gone by 60 minutes after cessation of the infusion. In dogs, however, aPC is antigenic and may result in anaphylaxis or in development of anti-aPC antibodies, which may predispose treated animals to thrombosis.[127] The required dose in dogs is also approximately 20-fold greater than humans to achieve the same anticoagulant effects.[126] These properties have hampered further investigation of aPC in dogs.

FFP contains PC and is the only available source of natural anticoagulant compounds for veterinary patients. Because of the extremely short half-life of aPC, there is unlikely to be any aPC contained in an FFP transfusion. FFP also contains molecules, such as protein C inhibitor, $\alpha2$-macroglobulin, and alpha 1-antitrypsin, that can scavenge aPC.

PLATELET TRANSFUSION

Platelet transfusions are generally not considered in human patients with DIC without active hemorrhage until the platelet count drops lower than 20,000 platelets/μL.[128,129] The cut-off number for transfusion is 50,000 platelets/μL in patients with ongoing hemorrhage, or in at-risk patients who must undergo invasive procedures.[128] Transfusions are generally of fresh platelet concentrates. There is no evidence in humans to show that transfusion to a platelet count higher than 50,000 platelets/μL has additional benefits. These guidelines seem reasonable for companion animals. There are several platelet products available for use in dogs, but many have not been extensively studied, even in healthy dogs.[130] Platelets may be transfused to dogs and cats via fresh whole blood transfusions if the blood is kept at room temperature and given within 4 hours of collection. Fresh whole blood may also be used to prepare PRP if the red blood cells are not required. Fresh canine platelet concentrates prepared by plateletpheresis may be available from some animal blood banks, and platelet concentrates are also available as a frozen dimethyl sulfoxide-stabilized product.[130] The recent availability of lyophilized canine platelets may be another treatment option for dogs who are experiencing hemorrhage secondary to thrombocytopenia.[130]

HEPARIN

The use of unfractionated heparin (UFH) in human patients with DIC is controversial. Although intuitively logical for slowing the consumptive aspects of DIC and minimizing the formation of microthrombi, the heparin molecule may also mitigate some of the antiinflammatory effects of endogenous compounds, such as AT. If the initial hypercoagulable phase of DIC could be reliably identified, heparin administration might be indicated to decrease thrombin production at that point. Heparin exerts an anticoagulant effect primarily by binding to AT, resulting in a 1000-fold increase in activity of the complex to inactivate coagulation factors Xa and IIa (among others).[131] Heparin binding to AT may interfere with the antiinflammatory effects of AT. For this reason, heparin is not indicated in patients with pending or actual DIC. A study in dogs showed that administration of heparin to healthy dogs caused a decrease in AT activity, presumably caused by increased participation in neutralizing procoagulant proteins.[118]

The use of heparin in human patients with DIC is indicated in those with overt thromboembolic disease (macrovascular thrombosis) and those at risk of extensive fibrin formation that could result in end-organ dysfunction (eg, renal failure from glomerular fibrin plugging). In addition, the presence of dermal or acral necrosis is a strong indication for heparin therapy.[132] Because heparin works in concert with AT, the activity may be diminished in patients with low AT activity. There has been no evidence to suggest that preincubation of FFP with plasma results in an increased heparin effect. Patients with thrombocytopenia or low levels of fibrinogen or those being treated concurrently with antiplatelet or other anticoagulant medications (eg, clopidogrel) may be at increased risk of bleeding with heparin therapy.[132]

Although the proinflammatory effects of unfractionated heparin are described, less information is available about whether the same can be expected of low molecular weight heparins (LMWH). There are few studies of LMWH as adjunctive therapy for DIC. One human study showed that dalteparin administration was more effective than unfractionated heparin at mitigating the thrombocytopenia and increase in FDP concentration associated with the development DIC in clinically ill humans.[133] Because LMWH also interacts with AT, similar proinflammatory effects may be seen, and the circulating AT levels will decrease over time with continued treatment at therapeutic levels. At least one study using dalteparin in rats showed attenuation of the inflammatory changes that occurred secondary to ischemia/reperfusion injury.[134] In this study, dalteparin did not affect endothelial prostacyclin production.

Human guidelines for dosing of heparin are based on anti-Xa activity (aXa) values, and vary depending on whether the drug is administered for prophylactic reasons or to treat a preexisting thrombus. The relationship between aPTT and aXa activity is variable, both with age as well as with laboratory equipment.[135] The recommendation for therapeutic UFH dosing in adults is target aXa levels between 0.35 and 0.7 U/mL. Patients with preexisting thrombi are more likely to benefit from intravenous dosing, rather than subcutaneous (SC) administration, at least when using UFH.[135] Prophylactic doses of UFH are 10% of the therapeutic levels and may be administered subcutaneously.[135] Guidelines for LMWH in both adult and pediatric humans target an aXa value of 0.5 to 1.0 U/mL for therapeutic uses and 0.1 to 0.3 U/mL for prophylaxis.[136] aXa activity is measured 4 to 6 hours after SC dosing.

In patients without an overt risk of hemorrhage, prophylactic doses of UFH or LMWH may be indicated for prevention of venous thromboembolism.[129] A low dose of UFH administered as an IV constant rate infusion (5–10 U/kg/h) for prophylaxis for venous thromboembolism has been advocated in human patients who have a concurrent bleeding risk, such as those with DIC.[129] Despite these recommendations, there are no clinical randomized, controlled trials in human medicine that demonstrate that the use of heparin in patients with DIC improves clinical outcome.[129] No studies have been done in veterinary species using these lower prophylactic doses of heparin.

Heparin has been administered to dogs using a wide variety of dosing regimens and is usually dose adjusted using the aPTT, with a goal of extending the aPTT 1.5 to 2.0 times the mean normal or baseline value.[101] These guidelines are derived from early human recommendations.[135] Just as in human medicine, the relationship of the aPTT to the actual aXa value is not easily predicted, and is likely variable based on the route of administration, individual patient, and clinical laboratory methodology.[137,138] The actual amount of circulating heparin is most accurately monitored by measuring anti-Xa activity levels in plasma,[139] although viscoelastic coagulation monitoring may provide another option if correlations with aXa values can be established.[140,141] In some canine studies, 200 U/kg of UFH administered subcutaneously to beagle dogs resulted in a peak mean aXa activity of 0.56 ± 0.2 U/mL approximately 4 hours after dosing. Another study using the same UFH dose in mixed-breed dogs achieved a peak mean aXa of 0.1 U/mL (range <0.1–0.5 U/mL) at 3 hours after a single dose. After 3 days of UFH administration to dogs at 200 U/kg subcutaneously every 8 hours, peak median aXa was 0.4 U/mL (range 0.2–0.65 U/mL).[137] A similar range was achieved in 6 healthy dogs given 300 U/kg of UFH subcutaneously every 8 hours for 3 days (0.4–0.6 U/mL, except for one dog who remained at 0.1 U/mL).[141] Studies in dogs with IMHA have shown that the administration of UFH at a dose of 300 U/kg subcutaneously every 6 hours resulted in therapeutic (ie, >0.35 U/mL) aXa levels in 31% of dogs (5/16) after 14 hours of therapy.[101] In this study and others, a significant correlation between aXa levels and aPTT was noted,[101,142] whereas this has not been the case in others.[137] In animals with acute inflammation, higher doses of UFH may be necessary to allow for nonspecific binding of the heparin molecules.[101] Another study in dogs in an intensive care unit noted hemorrhage in 4 of 6 dogs exposed to a high-dose UFH (900 U/kg/d, IV) protocol, whereas a lower dose (300 U/kg/d, IV) failed to achieve consistent aXa values.[143] Dosage studies in cats have been limited, but a dose of 250 U/kg UFH subcutaneously every 6 hours for 5 days resulted in aXa values in the therapeutic range (0.35–0.7 U/mL) in most cats for the majority of the study.[144] There was also a significant correlation between aPTT times and aXa values in the cats receiving UFH.[144] It is unclear if the target anti-Xa recommendations from human medicine can be transferred directly to veterinary patients, and prospective studies are warranted.

LMWH has become more popular in recent years, however, the optimal dose and drug for use in veterinary species is still undecided. In dogs with thromboplastin-induced DIC, dalteparin given as an IV CRI targeted to achieve aXa concentrations of 0.6 to 0.9 U/mL attenuated the hematologic changes associated with DIC.[145] A recent study of enoxaparin administered to dogs at a dose of 0.8 mg/kg subcutaneously every 6 hours indicated reliable aXa values more than 0.5 U/mL for the 36-hour dosing period.[146] A group of dogs in an intensive care unit setting who received dalteparin (100 U/kg subcutaneously every 12 hours) failed to achieve aXa values greater than 0.5 U/mL.[143] Another study of dalteparin in dogs using 150 U/kg subcutaneously every 8 hours showed a more reliable dose response.[147] Dalteparin given at 100 U/kg subcutaneously every 12 hours to cats also failed to reliably achieve target aXa values.[148] These results are consistent with another pharmacologic study, which predicted an effective dose of dalteparin, 150 IU/kg SC every 4 hours or enoxaparin, 1.5 mg/kg SC every 6 hours, to reliably achieve target aXa levels in healthy cats.[144]

ADDITIONAL THERAPY

In patients with DIC subsequent to hepatic or gastrointestinal disease, where there may be an absolute deficiency of vitamin K, this vitamin may be supplemented parenterally. This therapy may be especially relevant in cats. Vitamin K may be given to these patients at a dosage of 1 to 2 mg/kg subcutaneously every 24 hours.

In general, there is no indication for the use of antifibrinolytic agents in the treatment of DIC. In rare cases where the inciting cause may be hyperfibrinolysis leading to further consumptive coagulopathy, drugs, such as α amino caproic acid or tranexamic acid, may be indicated. To the authors' knowledge, this is a rare event, although the postoperative quasi-DIC hemorrhagic syndrome recognized in some greyhounds may be a result of enhanced fibrinolysis and may merit treatment in this manner.[149]

REFERENCES

1. Ivanyi B, Thoenes W. Microvascular injury and repair in acute human bacterial pyelonephritis. Virchows Arch A Pathol Anat Histopathol 1987;411:257–65.
2. Levi M, ten Cate H, van der Poll T, et al. Pathogenesis of disseminated intravascular coagulation in sepsis. JAMA 1993;270:975–9.
3. Rangel-Frausto MS, Pittet D, Costigan M, et al. The natural history of the systemic inflammatory response syndrome (SIRS). A prospective study. JAMA 1995;273:117–23.

4. Gando S, Kameue T, Nanzaki S, et al. Disseminated intravascular coagulation is a frequent complication of systemic inflammatory response syndrome. Thromb Haemost 1996;75:224–8.

5. Gando S, Kameue T, Matsuda N, et al. Combined activation of coagulation and inflammation has an important role in multiple organ dysfunction and poor outcome after severe trauma. Thromb Haemost 2002;88:943–9.

6. Gando S, Kameue T, Matsuda N, et al. Serial changes in neutrophil-endothelial activation markers during the course of sepsis associated with disseminated intravascular coagulation. Thromb Res 2005;116:91–100.

7. Fourrier F, Chopin C, Goudemand J, et al. Septic shock, multiple organ failure, and disseminated intravascular coagulation. Compared patterns of antithrombin III, protein C, and protein S deficiencies. Chest 1992;101:816–23.

8. Gando S. Microvascular thrombosis and multiple organ dysfunction syndrome. Crit Care Med 2010;38:S35–42.

9. Levi M, van der Poll T, ten Cate H. Tissue factor in infection and severe inflammation. Semin Thromb Hemost 2006;32:33–9.

10. Monroe DM, Hoffman M. What does it take to make the perfect clot? Arterioscler Thromb Vasc Biol 2006;26:41–8.

11. Esmon CT. Possible involvement of cytokines in diffuse intravascular coagulation and thrombosis. Baillieres Best Pract Res Clin Haematol 1999;12:343–59.

12. Levi M, Ten Cate H. Disseminated intravascular coagulation. N Engl J Med 1999;341:586–92.

13. Levi M, van der Poll T, ten Cate H, et al. The cytokine-mediated imbalance between coagulant and anticoagulant mechanisms in sepsis and endotoxaemia. Eur J Clin Invest 1997;27:3–9.

14. Morrissey JH. Tissue factor: a key molecule in hemostatic and nonhemostatic systems. Int J Hematol 2004;79:103–8.

15. Rauch U, Bonderman D, Bohrmann B, et al. Transfer of tissue factor from leukocytes to platelets is mediated by CD15 and tissue factor. Blood 2000; 96:170–5.

16. Eilertsen KE, Osterud B. The role of blood cells and their microparticles in blood coagulation. Biochem Soc Trans 2005;33:418–22.

17. Levi M, van der Poll T, Buller HR. Bidirectional relation between inflammation and coagulation. Circulation 2004;109:2698–704.

18. Eckle I, Seitz R, Egbring R, et al. Protein C degradation in vitro by neutrophil elastase. Biol Chem Hoppe Seyler 1991;372:1007–13.

19. Mesters RM, Helterbrand J, Utterback BG, et al. Prognostic value of protein C concentrations in neutropenic patients at high risk of severe septic complications. Crit Care Med 2000;28:2209–16.

20. Faust SN, Levin M, Harrison OB, et al. Dysfunction of endothelial protein C activation in severe meningococcal sepsis. N Engl J Med 2001;345:408–16.

21. Song D, Ye X, Xu H, et al. Activation of endothelial intrinsic NF-{kappa}B pathway impairs protein C anticoagulation mechanism and promotes coagulation in endotoxemic mice. Blood 2009;114:2521–9.

22. Esmon CT. The endothelial cell protein C receptor. Thromb Haemost 2000;83: 639–43.

23. Creasey AA, Reinhart K. Tissue factor pathway inhibitor activity in severe sepsis. Crit Care Med 2001;29:S126–9.

24. Abraham E, Reinhart K, Opal S, et al. Efficacy and safety of tifacogin (recombinant tissue factor pathway inhibitor) in severe sepsis: a randomized controlled trial. JAMA 2003;290:238–47.

25. Shibayama Y. Sinusoidal circulatory disturbance by microthrombosis as a cause of endotoxin-induced hepatic injury. J Pathol 1987;151:315–21.

26. Hewett JA, Jean PA, Kunkel SL, et al. Relationship between tumor necrosis factor-alpha and neutrophils in endotoxin-induced liver injury. Am J Physiol 1993;265:G1011–5.

27. Barbui T, Falanga A. Disseminated intravascular coagulation in acute leukemia. Semin Thromb Hemost 2001;27:593–604.

28. Sauaia A, Moore FA, Moore EE, et al. Epidemiology of trauma deaths: a reassessment. J Trauma 1995;38:185–93.

29. Stewart RM, Myers JG, Dent DL, et al. Seven hundred fifty-three consecutive deaths in a level I trauma center: the argument for injury prevention. J Trauma 2003;54:66–70 [discussion: 70–1].

30. Simpson SA, Syring R, Otto CM. Severe blunt trauma in dogs: 235 cases (1997–2003). J Vet Emerg Crit Care 2009;19:588–602.

31. Hess JR, Brohi K, Dutton RP, et al. The coagulopathy of trauma: a review of mechanisms. J Trauma 2008;65:748–54.

32. Smart L, Jandrey KE, Kass PH, et al. The effect of Hetastarch (670/0.75) in vivo on platelet closure time in the dog. J Vet Emerg Crit Care 2009;19:444–9.

33. Sohal AS, Gangji AS, Crowther MA, et al. Uremic bleeding: pathophysiology and clinical risk factors. Thromb Res 2006;118:417–22.

34. Mischke R, Schulze U. Studies on platelet aggregation using the Born method in normal and uraemic dogs. Vet J 2004;168:270–5.

35. Willis SE, Jackson ML, Meric SM, et al. Whole blood platelet aggregation in dogs with liver disease. Am J Vet Res 1989;50:1893–7.

36. Tripodi A, Mannucci PM. Abnormalities of hemostasis in chronic liver disease: reappraisal of their clinical significance and need for clinical and laboratory research. J Hepatol 2007;46:727–33.

37. Rao AK. Acquired qualitative platelets defects. In: Colman RW, Marder VJ, Clowes AW, et al, editors. Hemostasis and thrombosis 5th edition. 5th edition. St Louis (MO): Elsevier; 2005. p. 1045–51.

38. Levi M, de Jonge E, Meijers J. The diagnosis of disseminated intravascular coagulation. Blood Rev 2002;16:217–23.

39. Wiinberg B, Jensen AL, Johansson PI, et al. Development of a model based scoring system for diagnosis of canine disseminated intravascular coagulation with independent assessment of sensitivity and specificity. Vet J 2010;185(3):292–8.

40. Wiinberg B, Jensen AL, Johansson PI, et al. Thromboelastographic evaluation of hemostatic function in dogs with disseminated intravascular coagulation. J Vet Intern Med 2008;22:357–65.

41. Bateman SW, Mathews KA, Abrams-Ogg AC, et al. Diagnosis of disseminated intravascular coagulation in dogs admitted to an intensive care unit. J Am Vet Med Assoc 1999;215:798–804.

42. Bakhtiari K, Meijers JC, de Jonge E, et al. Prospective validation of the International Society of Thrombosis and Haemostasis scoring system for disseminated intravascular coagulation. Crit Care Med 2004;32:2416–21.

43. Taylor FB Jr, Toh CH, Hoots WK, et al. Towards definition, clinical and laboratory criteria, and a scoring system for disseminated intravascular coagulation. Thromb Haemost 2001;86:1327–30.

44. Mercer KW, Gail Macik B, Williams ME. Hematologic disorders in critically ill patients. Semin Respir Crit Care Med 2006;27:286–96.

45. Drews RE, Weinberger SE. Thrombocytopenic disorders in critically ill patients. Am J Respir Crit Care Med 2000;162:347–51.

46. Vanderschueren S, De Weerdt A, Malbrain M, et al. Thrombocytopenia and prognosis in intensive care. Crit Care Med 2000;28:1871–6.

47. Rebulla P, Finazzi G, Marangoni F, et al. The threshold for prophylactic platelet transfusions in adults with acute myeloid leukemia. Gruppo Italiano Malattie Ematologiche Maligne dell'Adulto. N Engl J Med 1997;337:1870–5.

48. Rebulla P. Revalidation of the clinical indications for the transfusion of platelet concentrates. Rev Clin Exp Hematol 2001;5:288–310.

49. Akca S, Haji-Michael P, de Mendonca A, et al. Time course of platelet counts in critically ill patients. Crit Care Med 2002;30:753–6.

50. de Laforcade AM, Freeman LM, Shaw SP, et al. Hemostatic changes in dogs with naturally occurring sepsis. J Vet Intern Med 2003;17:674–9.

51. Kristensen AT, Wiinberg B, Jessen LR, et al. Evaluation of human recombinant tissue factor-activated thromboelastography in 49 dogs with neoplasia. J Vet Intern Med 2008;22:140–7.

52. Sinnott VB, Otto CM. Use of thromboelastography in dogs with immune-mediated hemolytic anemia: 39 cases (2000–2008). J Vet Emerg Crit Care (San Antonio) 2009;19:484–8.

53. Donahue SM, Otto CM. Thromboelastography: a tool for measuring hypercoagulability, hypocoagulability, and fibrinolysis. J Vet Emerg Crit Care 2005;15:9–16.

54. Jaquith S, Brown AJ, Scott MA. The effect of hematocrit on canine thromboelastography. J Vet Emerg Crit Care 2009;19:A4.

55. Jaquith S, Scott MA, Brown AJ. The effect of platelet concentration on canine thromboelastography. 20th European College of Veterinary Internal Medicine Annual Congress. Toulouse (France), 2010.

56. Koenigshof AM, Scott MA, Sirivelu MP, et al. The effect of sample collection method on thromboelastography in healthy dogs. J Vet Emerg Crit Care 2009;19:A1–17.

57. Garcia-Pereira BL, Scott MA, Koenigshof AM, et al. Effect of venipuncture quality on thromboelastography in healthy dogs. J Vet Emerg Crit Care 2011, in press.

58. Ralph AG, Brainard BM, Babski DM, et al. The effect of storage temperature on thrombelastrography endpoints using citrated canine whole blood. Anaheim (CA): ACVIM Forum; 2010. p. 681.

59. Brainard BM, Abed JM, Koenig A. The effects of cytochalasin D and abciximab on hemostasis in canine whole blood assessed by thrombelastography and platelet function analyzer. J Vet Diag Invest 2011, in press.

60. Ralph AG, Koenig A, Pittman JR, et al. Effect of contact activation inhibition by corn trypsin inhibitor on TEG parameters in canine whole blood. J Vet Emerg Crit Care 2010;20:A6.

61. Puddu P, Puddu GM, Cravero E, et al. The involvement of circulating microparticles in inflammation, coagulation and cardiovascular diseases. Can J Cardiol 2010;26:140–5.

62. Horstman LL, Jy W, Jimenez JJ, et al. New horizons in the analysis of circulating cell-derived microparticles. Keio J Med 2004;53:210–30.

63. Combes V, Simon AC, Grau GE, et al. In vitro generation of endothelial microparticles and possible prothrombotic activity in patients with lupus anticoagulant. J Clin Invest 1999;104:93–102.

64. Chironi GN, Boulanger CM, Simon A, et al. Endothelial microparticles in diseases. Cell Tissue Res 2009;335:143–51.

65. Langer F, Spath B, Haubold K, et al. Tissue factor procoagulant activity of plasma microparticles in patients with cancer-associated disseminated intravascular coagulation. Ann Hematol 2008;87:451–7.

66. Soriano AO, Jy W, Chirinos JA, et al. Levels of endothelial and platelet microparticles and their interactions with leukocytes negatively correlate with organ dysfunction and predict mortality in severe sepsis. Crit Care Med 2005;33:2540–6.

67. Brooks MB, Randolph J, Warner K, et al. Evaluation of platelet function screening tests to detect platelet procoagulant deficiency in dogs with Scott syndrome. Vet Clin Pathol 2009;38:306–15.

68. Callan MB, Shofer FS, Wojenski C, et al. Chrono-lume and magnesium potentiate aggregation of canine but not human platelets in citrated platelet-rich plasma. Thromb Haemost 1998;80:176–80.

69. Forsythe LT, Jackson ML, Meric SM. Whole blood platelet aggregation in uremic dogs. Am J Vet Res 1989;50:1754–7.

70. Mischke R, Keidel A. Influence of platelet count, acetylsalicylic acid, von Willebrand's disease, coagulopathies, and haematocrit on results obtained using a platelet function analyser in dogs. Vet J 2003;165:43–52.

71. Callan MB, Giger U. Assessment of a point-of-care instrument for identification of primary hemostatic disorders in dogs. Am J Vet Res 2001;62:652–8.

72. Favaloro EJ, Facey D, Henniker A. Use of a novel platelet function analyzer (PFA-100) with high sensitivity to disturbances in von Willebrand factor to screen for von Willebrand's disease and other disorders. Am J Hematol 1999;62: 165–74.

73. Hayward CP, Harrison P, Cattaneo M, et al. Platelet function analyzer (PFA)-100 closure time in the evaluation of platelet disorders and platelet function. J Thromb Haemost 2006;4:312–9.

74. Moritz A, Walcheck BK, Weiss DJ. Evaluation of flow cytometric and automated methods for detection of activated platelets in dogs with inflammatory disease. Am J Vet Res 2005;66:325–9.

75. Tarnow I, Kristensen AT, Krogh AK, et al. Effects of physiologic agonists on canine whole blood flow cytometry assays of leukocyte-platelet aggregation and platelet activation. Vet Immunol Immunopathol 2008;123:345–52.

76. Weiss DJ, Brazzell JL. Detection of activated platelets in dogs with primary immune-mediated hemolytic anemia. J Vet Intern Med 2006;20:682–6.

77. de Laforcade AM, Rozanski EA, Freeman LM, et al. Serial evaluation of protein C and antithrombin in dogs with sepsis. J Vet Intern Med 2008;22:26–30.

78. Kuzi S, Segev G, Haruvi E, et al. Plasma antithrombin activity as a diagnostic and prognostic indicator in dogs: a retrospective study of 149 dogs. J Vet Intern Med 2010;24(3):587–96.

79. Scott-Moncrieff JC, Treadwell NG, McCullough SM, et al. Hemostatic abnormalities in dogs with primary immune-mediated hemolytic anemia. J Am Anim Hosp Assoc 2001;37:220–7.

80. Otto CM, Rieser TM, Brooks MB, et al. Evidence of hypercoagulability in dogs with parvoviral enteritis. J Am Vet Med Assoc 2000;217:1500–4.

81. Lorente JA, Garcia-Frade LJ, Landin L, et al. Time course of hemostatic abnormalities in sepsis and its relation to outcome. Chest 1993;103:1536–42.

82. Griffin A, Callan MB, Shofer FS, et al. Evaluation of a canine D-dimer point-of-care test kit for use in samples obtained from dogs with disseminated intravascular coagulation, thromboembolic disease, and hemorrhage. Am J Vet Res 2003;64:1562–9.

83. Nelson OL, Andreasen C. The utility of plasma D-dimer to identify thromboembolic disease in dogs. J Vet Intern Med 2003;17:830–4.

84. Stokol T, Brooks MB, Erb HN, et al. D-dimer concentrations in healthy dogs and dogs with disseminated intravascular coagulation. Am J Vet Res 2000;61:393–8.

85. Stansbury LG, Dutton RP, Stein DM, et al. Controversy in trauma resuscitation: do ratios of plasma to red blood cells matter? Transfus Med Rev 2009;23:255–65.
86. Weatherton LK, Streeter EM. Evaluation of fresh frozen plasma administration in dogs with pancreatitis: 77 cases (1995–2005). J Vet Emerg Crit Care 2009;19:617–22.
87. Leese T, Holliday M, Watkins M, et al. A multicentre controlled clinical trial of high-volume fresh frozen plasma therapy in prognostically severe acute pancreatitis. Ann R Coll Surg Engl 1991;73:207–14.
88. Boller EM, Otto CM. Septic shock. In: Silverstein DC, Hopper K, editors. Small animal critical care medicine. St Louis (MO): Saunders Elsevier; 2009. p. 459–63.
89. Hoenhaus AE. Blood transfusion and blood substitutes. In: DiBartola SP, editor. Fluid, electrolyte, and acid-base disorders in small animal practice. 3rd edition. St Louis (MO): Saunders Elsevier; 2006. p. 567–83.
90. Logan JC, Callan MB, Drew K, et al. Clinical indications for use of fresh frozen plasma in dogs: 74 dogs (October through December 1999). J Am Vet Med Assoc 2001;218:1449–55.
91. Snow SJ, Ari Jutkowitz L, Brown AJ. Trends in plasma transfusion at a veterinary teaching hospital: 308 patients (1996–1998 and 2006–2008). J Vet Emerg Crit Care 2010;20(4):441–5.
92. Estrin MA, Wehausen CE, Jessen CR, et al. Disseminated intravascular coagulation in cats. J Vet Intern Med 2006;20:1334–9.
93. Mueller MM, Bomke B, Seifried E. Fresh frozen plasma in patients with disseminated intravascular coagulation or in patients with liver diseases. Thromb Res 2002;107(Suppl 1):S9–17.
94. Dara SI, Rana R, Afessa B, et al. Fresh frozen plasma transfusion in critically ill medical patients with coagulopathy. Crit Care Med 2005;33:2667–71.
95. Stokol T, Parry B. Efficacy of fresh-frozen plasma and cryoprecipitate in dogs with von Willebrand's disease or hemophilia A. J Vet Intern Med 1998;12:84–92.
96. Brownlee L, Wardrop KJ, Sellon RK, et al. Use of a prestorage leukoreduction filter effectively removes leukocytes from canine whole blood while preserving red blood cell viability. J Vet Intern Med 2000;14:412–7.
97. Brainard BM, Alwood AJ, Kushner LI, et al. Postoperative pulmonary complications in dogs undergoing laparotomy: anesthetic and perioperative factors. J Vet Emerg Crit Care 2006;16:184–91.
98. Toy P, Gajic O. Transfusion-related acute lung injury. Anesth Analg 2004;99: 1623–4.
99. Levi M, van der Poll T. Inflammation and coagulation. Crit Care Med 2010;38:S26–34.
100. Ostrovsky L, Woodman RC, Payne D, et al. Antithrombin III prevents and rapidly reverses leukocyte recruitment in ischemia/reperfusion. Circulation 1997;96: 2302–10.
101. Breuhl EL, Moore G, Brooks MB, et al. A prospective study of unfractionated heparin therapy in dogs with primary immune-mediated hemolytic anemia. J Am Anim Hosp Assoc 2009;45:125–33.
102. Cheng T, Mathews KA, Abrams-Ogg AC, et al. Relationship between assays of inflammation and coagulation: a novel interpretation of the canine activated clotting time. Can J Vet Res 2009;73:97–102.
103. Thomas JS, Green RA. Clotting times and antithrombin III activity in cats with naturally developing diseases: 85 cases (1984–1994). J Am Vet Med Assoc 1998;213:1290–5.
104. Brazzell JL, Borjesson DL. Evaluation of plasma antithrombin activity and D-dimer concentration in populations of healthy cats, clinically ill cats, and cats with cardiomyopathy. Vet Clin Pathol 2007;36:79–84.

105. Rivera Ramirez PA, Deniz A, Wirth W, et al. Antithrombin III activity in health cats and its changes in selected disease. Berl Munch Tierarztl Wochenschr 1997;110:440–4.

106. Welles EG, Boudreaux MK, Crager CS, et al. Platelet function and antithrombin, plasminogen, and fibrinolytic activities in cats with heart disease. Am J Vet Res 1994;55:619–27.

107. Stokol T, Brooks M, Rush JE, et al. Hypercoagulability in cats with cardiomyopathy. J Vet Intern Med 2008;22:546–52.

108. Mammen EF. Antithrombin: its physiological importance and role in DIC. Semin Thromb Hemost 1998;24:19–25.

109. Warren BL, Eid A, Singer P, et al. Caring for the critically ill patient. High-dose antithrombin III in severe sepsis: a randomized controlled trial. JAMA 2001; 286:1869–78.

110. Hoffmann JN, Wiedermann CJ, Juers M, et al. Benefit/risk profile of high-dose antithrombin in patients with severe sepsis treated with and without concomitant heparin. Thromb Haemost 2006;95:850–6.

111. Kienast J, Juers M, Wiedermann CJ, et al. Treatment effects of high-dose antithrombin without concomitant heparin in patients with severe sepsis with or without disseminated intravascular coagulation. J Thromb Haemost 2006;4:90–7.

112. Lavrentieva A, Kontakiotis T, Bitzani M, et al. The efficacy of antithrombin administration in the acute phase of burn injury. Thromb Haemost 2008;100:286–90.

113. Horie S, Ishii H, Kazama M. Heparin-like glycosaminoglycan is a receptor for antithrombin III-dependent but not for thrombin-dependent prostacyclin production in human endothelial cells. Thromb Res 1990;59:895–904.

114. Zeerleder S, Hack CE, Wuillemin WA. Disseminated intravascular coagulation in sepsis. Chest 2005;128:2864–75.

115. Hoffmann JN, Vollmar B, Laschke MW, et al. Adverse effect of heparin on antithrombin action during endotoxemia: microhemodynamic and cellular mechanisms. Thromb Haemost 2002;88:242–52.

116. Spiess BD. Treating heparin resistance with antithrombin or fresh frozen plasma. Ann Thorac Surg 2008;85:2153–60.

117. Thompson MF, Scott-Moncrieff JC, Brooks MB. Effect of a single plasma transfusion on thromboembolism in 13 dogs with primary immune-mediated hemolytic anemia. J Am Anim Hosp Assoc 2004;40:446–54.

118. Rozanski EA, Hughes D, Scotti M, et al. The effect of heparin and fresh frozen plasma on plasma antithrombin III activity, prothrombin time and activated partial thromboplastin time in critically ill dogs. J Vet Emerg Crit Care 2001;11:15–21.

119. Mammen EF, Miyakawa T, Phillips TF, et al. Human antithrombin concentrates and experimental disseminated intravascular coagulation. Semin Thromb Hemost 1985;11:373–83.

120. Woodman RC, Teoh D, Payne D, et al. Thrombin and leukocyte recruitment in endotoxemia. Am J Physiol Heart Circ Physiol 2000;279:H1338–45.

121. Grey ST, Tsuchida A, Hau H, et al. Selective inhibitory effects of the anticoagulant activated protein C on the responses of human mononuclear phagocytes to LPS, IFN-gamma, or phorbol ester. J Immunol 1994;153:3664–72.

122. Bernard GR, Vincent JL, Laterre PF, et al. Efficacy and safety of recombinant human activated protein C for severe sepsis. N Engl J Med 2001;344:699–709.

123. Vincent JL, Angus DC, Artigas A, et al. Effects of drotrecogin alfa (activated) on organ dysfunction in the PROWESS trial. Crit Care Med 2003;31:834–40.

124. Dhainaut JF, Yan SB, Joyce DE, et al. Treatment effects of drotrecogin alfa (activated) in patients with severe sepsis with or without overt disseminated intravascular coagulation. J Thromb Haemost 2004;2:1924–33.

125. Wiedermann CJ, Kaneider NC. A meta-analysis of controlled trials of recombinant human activated protein C therapy in patients with sepsis. BMC Emerg Med 2005;5:7.

126. Jackson CV, Bailey BD, Shetler TJ. Pharmacological profile of recombinant, human activated protein C (LY203638) in a canine model of coronary artery thrombosis. J Pharmacol Exp Ther 2000;295:967–71.

127. Eli Lilly and Co. Data on File.

128. Ten Cate H. Thrombocytopenia: one of the markers of disseminated intravascular coagulation. Pathophysiol Haemost Thromb 2003;33:413–6.

129. Levi M, Toh CH, Thachil J, et al. Guidelines for the diagnosis and management of disseminated intravascular coagulation. British Committee for Standards in Haematology. Br J Haematol 2009;145:24–33.

130. Callan MB, Appleman EH, Sachais BS. Canine platelet transfusions. J Vet Emerg Crit Care 2009;19:401–15.

131. Pratt CW, Church FC. Antithrombin: structure and function. Semin Hematol 1991;28:3–9.

132. Marder VJ, Feinstein DI, Colman RW, et al. Consumptive thrombohemorrhagic disorders. In: Colman RW, Hirsh J, Marder VJ, et al, editors. Hemostasis and thrombosis: basic principles and clinical practice. 5th edition. Philadelphia (PA): Lippincott Williams & Wilkins; 2005. p. 1023–63.

133. Sakuragawa N, Hasegawa H, Maki M, et al. Clinical evaluation of low-molecular-weight heparin (FR-860) on disseminated intravascular coagulation (DIC)– a multicenter co-operative double-blind trial in comparison with heparin. Thromb Res 1993;72:475–500.

134. Harada N, Okajima K, Uchiba M. Dalteparin, a low molecular weight heparin, attenuates inflammatory responses and reduces ischemia-reperfusion-induced liver injury in rats. Crit Care Med 2006;34:1883–91.

135. Hirsh J, Bauer KA, Donati MB, et al. Parenteral anticoagulants: American College of Chest Physicians Evidence-Based Clinical Practice Guidelines (8th Edition). Chest 2008;133:141S–59S.

136. Monagle P, Chalmers E, Chan A, et al. Antithrombotic therapy in neonates and children: American College of Chest Physicians Evidence-Based Clinical Practice Guidelines (8th Edition). Chest 2008;133:887S–968S.

137. Pittman JR, Koenig A, Brainard BM. The effect of unfractionated heparin on thrombelastographic analysis in healthy dogs. J Vet Emerg Crit Care 2010;20(2):216–23.

138. Spinler SA, Wittkowsky AK, Nutescu EA, et al. Anticoagulation monitoring part 2: unfractionated heparin and low-molecular-weight heparin. Ann Pharmacother 2005;39:1275–85.

139. Brooks MB. Evaluation of a chromogenic assay to measure the factor Xa inhibitory activity of unfractionated heparin in canine plasma. Vet Clin Pathol 2004;33:208–14.

140. Jessen LR, Wiinberg B, Jensen AL, et al. In vitro heparinization of canine whole blood with low molecular weight heparin (dalteparin) significantly and dose-dependently prolongs heparinase-modified tissue factor-activated thromboelastography parameters and prothrombinase-induced clotting time. Vet Clin Pathol 2008;37:363–72.

141. Babski DA, Brainard BM, Pittman JR, et al. Relationship of aXa and sonoclot parameters in dogs treated with unfractionated heparin. J Vet Emerg Crit Care 2010;20:A1.

142. Diquelou A, Barbaste C, Gabaig AM, et al. Pharmacokinetics and pharmacodynamics of a therapeutic dose of unfractionated heparin (200 U/kg) administered subcutaneously or intravenously to healthy dogs. Vet Clin Pathol 2005;34:237–42.

143. Scott KC, Hansen BD, DeFrancesco TC. Coagulation effects of low molecular weight heparin compared with heparin in dogs considered to be at risk for clinically significant venous thrombosis. J Vet Emerg Crit Care (San Antonio) 2009; 19:74–80.

144. Alwood AJ, Downend AB, Brooks MB, et al. Anticoagulant effects of low-molecular-weight heparins in healthy cats. J Vet Intern Med 2007;21:378–87.

145. Mischke R, Fehr M, Nolte I. Efficacy of low molecular weight heparin in a canine model of thromboplastin-induced acute disseminated intravascular coagulation. Res Vet Sci 2005;79:69–76.

146. Lunsford KV, Mackin AJ, Langston VC, et al. Pharmacokinetics of subcutaneous low molecular weight heparin (enoxaparin) in dogs. J Am Anim Hosp Assoc 2009;45:261–7.

147. Mischke RH, Schuttert C, Grebe SI. Anticoagulant effects of repeated subcutaneous injections of high doses of unfractionated heparin in healthy dogs. Am J Vet Res 2001;62:1887–91.

148. Vargo CL, Taylor SM, Carr A, et al. The effect of a low molecular weight heparin on coagulation parameters in healthy cats. Can J Vet Res 2009;73:132–6.

149. Lara-Garcia A, Couto CG, Iazbik MC, et al. Postoperative bleeding in retired racing greyhounds. J Vet Intern Med 2008;22:525–33.

Alterations of Drug Metabolism in Critically Ill Animals

Eileen S. Hackett, DVM, MS*, Daniel L. Gustafson, PhD

KEYWORDS

• Pharmacology • Pharmacokinetics
• Pharmacodynamics • Dogs

Pharmacotherapy in the critically ill presents many challenges. Illness may result in altered drug kinetics and pathophysiologic differences, altering pharmacodynamics. In addition, critical illness results from varied disease etiologies that may further affect goals of pharmacologic treatment. Animals of all ages, breeds, and species often present with acute disease requiring immediate therapy. Treatment may be complicated by underlying chronic disease and preexisting drug therapy. There are few well-controlled clinical trials in critically ill animals that evaluate alterations in drug metabolism. This article focuses on a review of pharmacologic principles that guide pharmacotherapy in the critical care setting, to improve the understanding of caregivers in basic processes governing dosing recommendations.

PHARMACOKINETICS

Pharmacokinetics play a key role in drug dose modification in the critically ill. Only through understanding specific pharmacokinetics principles is it possible to achieve the most rapid beneficial effect while minimizing adverse events. Pharmacokinetics is defined by the absorption, distribution, metabolism, and elimination of a drug, commonly referred to as ADME. Drug absorption is a critical process in drug dosing and determining the route of delivery. Regardless of administration route, drugs must transit biological membranes to enter the circulatory system and be systemically distributed. For intravenous administration, membrane crossing is accomplished via mechanical means. For oral, subcutaneous, intramuscular, and transdermal dose routes, absorption is a function of the concentration of drug in solution at the site of absorption, permeability, and the concentration gradient across membranes, as

The authors have nothing to disclose.
Department of Clinical Sciences, Colorado State University, 300 West Drake Road, Fort Collins, CO 80523, USA
* Corresponding author.
E-mail address: Eileen.Hackett@colostate.edu

demonstrated in the formula below where k_a is rate of absorption, P is drug permeability, and Gradient reflects the concentration difference between the site of absorption and the local blood.

$$k_a = [\text{Drug}]_{\text{solution}} \times P \times \text{Gradient}$$

Resulting conclusions from the relationships shown in this equation are that drug absorption rate is a function of drug dissolution if not given in solution (drug concentration), lipophilicity and ionization state (permeability), and the rate of perfusion at the site of administration, such that absorbed drug is quickly removed and a diffusion-driving concentration gradient maintained. Permeability and the maintenance of a concentration gradient are relatively consistent within a local drug depot, thus drug absorption from extravascular sites often occurs via a first-order rate. This can be described by an absorption rate constant (k_a) as long as the amount of drug in solution is not limiting. For oral drug dosing, complicating factors in absorption include transit time through the gastrointestinal (GI) tract, competing reactions with GI contents, metabolism by GI tissue, active transport from GI epithelium toward the gut lumen, and metabolism of absorbed drug by the liver due to portal blood outflow. Oral dosing can show limited exposure due to any of these factors, thus these competing processes temper the amount of drug traversing the gastrointestinal epithelium and reaching the systemic circulation. This situation differs in parenteral sites, where drug absorption is often simply a function of permeability across cellular membranes and access to the circulation. Bioavailability (F) is the measure of drug absorption and exposure from extravascular sites. Bioavailability represents simply the drug exposure (area under the curve; AUC) following the extravascular dose in comparison to drug exposure following intravenous (IV) dosing, and is determined by:

$$F = \frac{\text{AUC}_{\text{extravascular}} \times \text{Dose}_{\text{IV}}}{\text{AUC}_{\text{IV}} \times \text{Dose}_{\text{extravascular}}}$$

The movement of drug from the blood to tissues is termed distribution and occurs in perfusion-limited or diffusion-limited manners. Drugs that readily cross biological membranes and where delivery to tissues is dependent only on the rate of delivery (ie, blood flow) are said to be perfusion-limited. The movement of drug into tissues is diffusion-limited when dependent on the movement of drug molecules from the blood into the tissue, with factors of facilitated transport and tissue properties affecting the rate and extent of drug uptake. Protein binding in the blood as well as in tissues is another component of drug distribution. Drug binding within the blood compartment can include binding to blood cellular components as well as proteins and lipoproteins within the plasma component. Albumin and α1-acid glycoprotein are the major plasma proteins responsible for drug binding. Protein binding within the blood can have a major impact on drug distribution, metabolism, and elimination depending on the degree and extent of the drug-protein interaction. Drug plasma concentrations are usually reported as total drug (protein bound and unbound), thus protein binding may be a variability factor associated with plasma drug levels and drug effects. Drug that is protein bound in the plasma has limited tissue distribution, cannot elicit a pharmacodynamic response, and will not be metabolized or eliminated. The dynamic of drug movement from a bound to unbound state and how rapid this free drug distributes to tissues resulting in binding to effector sites, or metabolism and elimination, dictates drug action. Therefore, pharmacologically relevant descriptions of drug distribution include the common pharmacokinetic parameter Volume of Distribution (V_d), describing the relationship between amount of drug in the body and the concentration in the plasma, as well as protein-binding descriptors such as the fraction of drug unbound in the plasma (f_u).

The conversion of a drug molecule into another molecular entity is termed drug metabolism and can result in the formation of inactive, toxic, and active metabolites, further complicating the pharmacology of given agents. The liver is the major metabolizing organ, with other tissues contributing depending on the nature of the metabolizing system and its physiologic distribution. Metabolism in a general sense is viewed as a mechanism of drug loss from the body, and this process generally follows saturation (Michaelis-Menten) kinetics described by the following equation, where V_{max} represents the maximal rate of metabolism and K_m is a measure of drug affinity for a specific enzymatic process.

$$\text{Rate of Metabolism} = \frac{V_{max} \times [\text{Drug}]}{K_m + [\text{Drug}]}$$

Most drug metabolism processes occurs within a range of drug concentrations far lower than the K_m for the metabolizing enzyme(s). Therefore, the rate of metabolism is proportional to drug concentration and follows a first-order rate described by the following equation, with the term V_{max}/K_m representing a constant whose resulting units are reciprocal time:

$$\text{Rate of Metabolism} = \frac{V_{max}}{K_m} \times [\text{Drug}]$$

In rare cases where the drug concentration is close to or greatly exceeds the K_m of a metabolizing enzyme, the rate of drug metabolism will not be dose-proportional and will result in either zero-order (Rate of metabolism = V_{max}) or saturation characteristics. In these cases where metabolizing enzymes systems are saturated and metabolism is not dose-proportional, the relationships between dose and drug exposure become nonlinear and difficult to predict.

Multiple metabolic pathways are often associated with the metabolism of an individual drug. Assuming no interaction between the metabolic pathways, the sum of the individual pathways will represent total drug metabolism. Drug metabolism can be a major point of drug interaction, as several factors, including drugs competing for the active site of a metabolizing enzyme and depletion of cofactors, can come into play. Induction of metabolizing enzymes can lead to proportional increases in the rate of drug metabolism. As drug metabolism is not necessarily synonymous with drug inactivation, metabolites may be active and potentially toxic. Metabolic activation and/or inactivation must be considered for a given drug's efficacy and toxicity.

Drug elimination is a catch-all phrase describing loss of drug from the plasma or serum. The major drug eliminating organs are the liver and the kidney, but drugs and drug metabolites can leave the body through other routes including exhaled air, sweat, saliva, and breast milk. For the majority of compounds, however, the urine and feces are the major route of elimination from the body. Metabolism and transport of drugs into the bile are components of hepatic elimination, therefore metabolizing enzymes (ie, P450, glucuronyl transferases, and so forth) and drug transporters (ie, ABC, OAT, OCT, and so forth) are involved. Drug transporters are also abundant in the gastrointestinal epithelium, and it is reasonable to assume that drugs can be directly eliminated from GI tissue into the feces. The complexity of drug elimination and transport within the hepatobiliary and gastrointestinal circulation, as well as the drug absorption properties associated with the GI tract, leads to the potential for drug cycling (enterohepatic cycling) within these tissues and buildup of drug and drug metabolites.

In renal elimination, transport of xenobiotics into the urine occurs by glomerular filtration and/or active transport. Drug accumulation in the urine results from both passive filtering at the glomerulus and active transport, primarily in the proximal tubule. Reabsorption tempers drug accumulation in the urine, as drugs with high permeability of biological membranes can reenter the circulation. Thus, renal elimination of highly lipophilic compounds is essentially limited to the urine concentration being equal to the plasma concentration. Drug metabolism overcomes this problem by adding functional groups, such as glucuronic acid, sulfate, or amino acids, decreasing membrane permeability and enhancing solubility. For many compounds, significant renal elimination is limited to their conjugated (glucuronide, sulfate, glutathione, and so forth) forms. Net renal elimination is summarized as:

Renal Elimination = Glomerular Filtration + Active Secretion − Reabsorption

Elimination half-life refers to the time necessary to reduce the pharmaceutical within the body by half. Factors affecting elimination half-life are represented by the following formula, where V_d is volume of distribution and CL is clearance:

Elimination half-life $T_{1/2} = (0.693 \times V_d)/CL$

Increases in drug clearance will reduce the elimination half-life, whereas increases in volume of distribution will increase the elimination half-life.

PHYSIOLOGIC ALTERATIONS IN CRITICAL ILLNESS THAT AFFECT DRUG DISPOSITION AND THERAPEUTIC RESPONSE
Renal

As previously stated, the kidneys are an important source of excretion of many drug compounds. Renal insufficiency can affect drug disposition, but not by clearance alone. Uremia-induced ileus can result in a lower rate of enteral drug absorption. Protein binding is typically diminished, due to both an accumulation of organic acids and structural change to the albumin molecule secondary to uremia. Volume of distribution may be altered, especially with those compounds that are acidic, highly protein bound, or ordinarily have a small volume of distribution. Clearance will be significantly lower for drugs in which greater than one-third is excreted unchanged in the urine.[1] Renal replacement therapy also affects drug clearance.

Renal insufficiency may be an acute or chronic underlying condition in the critically ill. There are multiple strategies to quantifying the degree of renal insufficiency. Estimation of glomerular filtration rate (GFR) is an approximation of renal filtration function. Calculation of endogenous creatinine clearance is a common method for estimation of GFR, and is typically calculated using a 12- or 24-hour timed urine collection.[2] Use of a 2-hour urine collection for calculation of creatinine clearance results in a reasonable correlation with 24-hour results, and may be more practical in the intensive care unit.[3] Creatinine clearance can be calculated using the following formula:

Creatinine Clearance = $U_{Cr} \cdot V/P_{Cr}$

where U_{Cr} is urine creatinine concentration, V is volume of urine produced over a timed collection in mL/min divided by body weight in kg, and P_{Cr} is serum creatinine concentration. The normal value in dogs and cats is 2 to 5 mL/min/kg^2.

Renal scintigraphy is an accurate method to estimate GFR in animals, though as specialized equipment, expertise, and licensing are required, this modality is not widely available in veterinary practices.[4] The most common estimation of renal function in small animal critical care is urine output, which normally should be between

1 and 2 mL/kg/h.[5] Age-related decrease in muscle mass may mask decline in renal function classically associated with elevations in creatinine. Hepatic insufficiency, associated with low serum creatinine, may also mask concurrent renal insufficiency.

Hepatic

As the liver is the body's most important site of drug biotransformation, liver injury can result in relevant changes in drug efficacy and clearance.[1,6] Alterations in hepatic blood flow and enzyme function contribute to altered drug disposition in critical illness.[7] Sources of liver injury common in the critically ill include intoxication, ischemic injury, neoplasia, sepsis, and trauma.[1] Liver dysfunction can affect pharmacokinetics by changing volume of distribution. The effects on volume of distribution are complex and unpredictable. Volume of distribution is increased in cases with third spacing of fluids into the abdominal cavity or extremities, but decreased in cases with less protein synthesis and binding, resulting in increased clearance of unbound free drug. Lower protein synthesis can also limit tissue penetration of highly protein-bound drugs.[1] Oral bioavailability may be significantly higher with drugs that normally undergo extensive hepatic metabolism. Endotoxemia may directly impair hepatic enzymatic drug metabolism.[8] With hepatic dysfunction, drug dosage should be altered based on severity of liver damage, degree of hepatic drug elimination, extent of protein binding, and route of administration.[1] When possible, pharmacodynamic and therapeutic drug monitoring should be used to guide therapy.

While most agree that hepatic injury is prominent in critically ill patients with multiorgan dysfunction, quantification of the impact of hepatic disturbance is difficult. In patients with hepatic injury affecting 40% to greater than 90% of liver function, urea production, blood glucose regulation, and bilirubin elimination may be maintained, limiting clinicopathologic testing methods in quantitation of liver injury. Often veterinarians estimate the degree of liver injury based on albumin and factor synthesis, enzyme concentration, and histopathology. Probe drugs that undergo enzyme specific degradation can be used to evaluate alterations in hepatic drug metabolism.[9,10] A clear advantage of using probe drugs is that this allows a better understanding of the individual metabolic derangement related to critical illness. The decrease in activity of cytochrome P450 enzymes secondary to hepatic dysfunction is not uniform and difficult to predict,[6] further supporting the use of probe drug technology. Disadvantages of probe drug evaluation include the requirement of multiple blood samples and time-consuming laboratory analysis. A recently published approach mitigates disadvantages of probe drug analysis through use of a single compound, intravenous midazolam, followed by a single-measurement time point.[9] Results of this approach are promising. Further study with single-dose midazolam in critically ill human patients reveals the interrelationship between multiple body systems. Critically ill patients with acute kidney injury, defined as diminished estimated GFR, underwent a greater reduction in hepatic metabolism of midazolam than those with critical illness alone.

Gastrointestinal

Critical illness can have profound effects on gastrointestinal function. Not uncommonly, diminished intestinal perfusion, bowel wall edema, ileus, and increased intra-abdominal pressure (IAP) can result in alterations in gut absorptive function and motility.[1,11] Gastrointestinal dysfunction in critically ill animals may limit reliability of enteral medication absorption. Drug absorption by both passive diffusion and active transport is altered by systemic illness.[7] Despite this, enterally administered gastrointestinal protectants are often necessary to limit morbidity associated with alterations in mucosal blood flow and delayed return to enteral feeding. When enteral drugs are administered in the critically ill, a larger dose may be necessary to offset diminished bioavailability and result in therapeutic plasma concentrations. A secondary consideration with oral medications is the impact of presystemic hepatic metabolism or "first-pass" effect, which can be altered with both disease and concurrently administered drug interactions.[1] Despite the limitations of enteral medications in critical illness, preservation of flora and mucosal barrier health is improved when enteral nutrition is maintained.[11]

Cardiovascular

Sources of circulatory failure in the critically ill include congestive heart failure, severe trauma, and sepsis. Congestive heart failure has the capacity to alter multiple pharmacokinetic parameters of commonly administered drugs. These factors include diminished bioavailability due to bowel wall edema, hepatic congestion, and peripheral edema, altered volume of distribution due to tissue hypoperfusion and increased total body water, diminished biotransformation especially of flow-dependent drugs metabolized in the liver, and impaired renal excretion related to blood flow and GFR.[1] Less is known about the impact of sepsis and systemic inflammatory response syndrome on the disposition of drugs. Renal and hepatic blood flow may be disproportionately affected, resulting in greater organ impairment than that suspected by global hemodynamic measurement.[1] Large doses of intravenous fluids required to support blood pressure and tissue perfusion may result in dramatic increases in volume of distribution of drugs, justifying higher dosages.[12] Cardiac indices are often higher than normal in critical illness,[13,14] but significant myocardial depression can accompany health deterioration as illness progresses, contributing to multiple organ dysfunction syndrome.[15,16] Decreased circulation and organ function can contribute to decreased drug clearance and risk of toxicity of both parent drug and metabolites.

SPECIFIC DRUGS USED IN THE CRITICAL CARE SETTING
Benzodiazepines

Benzodiazepines consist of a combination of benzene and diazepine rings, and undergo glucuronidation, most with multiple active metabolites.[17] Relative rate of entry into the site of action of different benzodiazepine compounds, the central nervous system (CNS), is dependent on degree of lipid solubility.[17] Benzodiazepines produce sedation-hypnosis by potentiating inhibitory γ-aminobutyric acid A (GABA$_A$) receptor chloride channels.[17] These agents are most commonly used in critically ill animals for sedation and treatment of status epilepticus. Sedation is necessary to allow delivery of nursing care, improve compliance during mechanical ventilation, minimize the dose of anesthetic agents, and perform minor procedures.[18] Benzodiazepines most often used in veterinary medicine are diazepam, midazolam, lorazepam, and zolazepam (currently only available in combination with tiletamine in the drug Telazol). Cats have an intrinsically lower rate of glucuronidation than dogs, increasing elimination half-life and decreasing clearance of these compounds. In addition, hepatic failure has been reported following repeated oral administration of diazepam in cats, prompting caution when additional doses are necessary.[17] Hepatic dysfunction is a contraindication for use. Potent active metabolites of diazepam that require renal excretion may limit this drug's use in critically ill animals with renal insufficiency.[19] In such cases, lorazepam may be a preferable choice, as it does not have active metabolites. Disadvantages of lorazepam use include poor aqueous solubility and longer onset of action.[19] Midazolam is preferred for continuous-rate infusion (CRI) because of its short elimination half-life, lack of significant active metabolites, and aqueous solubility.[19] Daily interruption of sedative infusions can reduce total amount and duration of use, as well as decrease accumulation within peripheral tissues.[20] Regardless of the drug selected for sedation in the critically ill, the minimum dose resulting in the minimum depth of sedation appropriate should be used to avoid adverse events.[21] Degree of sedation should be evaluated frequently to maintain consistency. Overdose of benzodiazepines can result in disorientation, tremors, respiratory depression (decrease in tidal volume with increased respiratory rate, decrease in hypoxic ventilatory drive), and hypotension, and are most often treated with supportive care and the specific antagonist flumazenil.[17–19]

Opioids

Opioids are natural opium derivatives or synthetic compounds that affect opiate receptors and provide analgesia.[22] Opioids undergo high hepatic extraction and therefore rely primarily on maintenance of hepatic blood flow for clearance. Dose adjustments are therefore necessary in cardiogenic shock states and other low-flow shock states.[23] Opioid glucuronide metabolite clearance is decreased with renal impairment, though metabolite accumulation does not have clinical consequences in animals.[22] Analgesia effects of opioids occur through stimulation of μ, κ, or δ receptors in the CNS.[23] Provision of analgesia in critically ill animals is a key component of veterinary care, addressing both presenting complaint and procedural interventions. Untreated pain in the critically ill can result in increased endogenous catecholamine activity, myocardial ischemia, hypermetabolic states, anxiety, and adverse outcomes.[18,23,24] Opioids most often used in critically ill animals are morphine, hydromorphone, methadone, and fentanyl. Opioid use has been associated with alterations in temperature regulation by a direct effect on the hypothalamus thermoregulatory center, resulting in hypothermia in dogs and hyperthermia in cats.[25–28] Overdose of opioids can result in dysphoria and respiratory depression, and can be treated with supportive care and the specific antagonist naloxone.[22] Respiratory depression is dose dependent and is mediated by μ-2 receptors in the medulla.[18] Opioids should be used with caution in animals with head trauma, as respiratory depression can lead to increased blood carbon dioxide, cerebral vasodilation, and exacerbation of cerebral edema.[22] Opioid-induced CNS excitation can be treated with benzodiazepines or barbiturates.[29]

Propofol

Propofol is an alkyl-phenol derivative that is highly lipid soluble and undergoes high hepatic extraction.[30,31] Drug clearance is slower in greyhounds and geriatric dogs, due to population differences in metabolism.[32–34] Propofol produces hypnosis by potentiating inhibitory $GABA_A$ receptor chloride channels.[35] It is used most commonly in critically ill animals for sedation, anesthesia, and treatment of status epilepticus. One important limitation is the high interindividual variability commonly observed in response to propofol use in the critically ill. For this reason, further study in special populations has been endorsed to discover methods to improve predictability.[36] Disease severity has been identified as a major determinant of propofol pharmacodynamics.[37] Critically ill patients required a downward titration of propofol, and those with cardiac failure required a 38% reduction in dose.[37] Unfortunately, in a study performed in critically ill human patients, clearance of propofol, though influenced by liver blood flow, did not correlate with cardiac output or cardiac index, negating the use of cardiac indices for rational dose adjustment.[36] It is interesting that a wide range of liver blood flow was observed in these critically ill patients, which may in part elucidate the difficulty in predicting kinetics of highly extracted drugs in this special population.[36] Severe cardiovascular and respiratory depression can occur with overdoses of propofol, though with supportive treatment duration is short.[31]

Antibacterials

Antimicrobial drugs are commonly prescribed in the critically ill.[12] Optimizing antibiotic therapy is of primary importance in critically ill animals with infections. In vivo efficacy is determined in large part by the pharmacokinetic and pharmacodynamic properties of specific antimicrobial agents and the translation of these properties in the clinical situation.[12] Pharmacokinetics of hydrophilic antibiotics, such as aminoglycosides, β-lactams, and carbapenems, are most dramatically affected by increases in volume of distribution and alterations in drug clearance relative to creatinine clearance.[38] Increase in volume of distribution, proportional to illness severity, will result in a lower maximum concentration and diminished efficacy of aminoglycosides without appropriate dose adjustment.[39] Because of the narrow therapeutic index of this drug, therapeutic drug monitoring should accompany dose adjustment. Circumstances where volume of distribution is directly affected in the critical care unit are many. Volume of distribution is influenced by intravenous fluid therapy, total parental nutrition, indwelling surgical drains, endotoxemia, mechanical ventilation, hypoalbuminemia, severe burns, and pleural and peritoneal effusion.[12,38] Lipophilic antibiotics, such as fluoroquinolones and macrolides, are less affected by alterations in volume of distribution, but may undergo alterations in clearance secondary to critical illness.[38] Highly protein-bound antibiotics, such as ceftriaxone, can have 100% greater clearance and 90% greater volume of distribution in hypoalbuminemic states.[40]

Clinicians must adjust dosing regimens appropriately to maximize response rate and ensure a favorable outcome. With traditional bolus dosing of β-lactam and carbapenem time-dependent antibiotics, concentrations decrease to low levels between doses.[41] Recent studies indicate improved clinical cures if levels are consistently maintained above the minimum inhibitory concentration.[42] To achieve this, treatment can be adjusted by using more frequent dosing, extended infusions, or CRI.[43] Despite the large therapeutic window of these classes of antibiotics, clinicians may consider reducing either dose or frequency in moderate to severe renal dysfunction.[38]

Tissue penetration is a critical element in the treatment of bacterial sepsis. Recently, microdialysis technology has allowed evaluation of antibiotic pharmacokinetics within target tissues.[44] In human critically ill patients with septic shock, antibiotic penetration into tissues is significantly impaired, nearly 5 to 10 times less than that of healthy volunteers.[45–47] High dosing of antibiotics may be necessary in patients with sepsis and septic shock in order to counteract severe limitations in microvascular perfusion.

SUMMARY

Principles of pharmacology guide safe and effective use of pharmaceuticals in critically ill animals. Though not common in veterinary medicine, inclusion of a pharmacologist in the critical care team may assist in rational dose adjustment and minimization of adverse drug events. Dosing recommendations should be based on known drug characteristics, as well as clinical trials in special populations.

REFERENCES

1. Krishnan V, Murray P. Pharmacologic issues in the critically ill. Clin Chest Med 2003;24(4):671–88.

2. DiBartola SP. Clinical approach and laboratory evaluation of renal disease. In: Ettinger SJ, Feldman EC, editors. Textbook of veterinary internal medicine. 7th edition. St Louis (MO): Saunders Elsevier; 2010. p. 1955–69.
3. Herrera-Gutierrez ME, Seller-Perez G, Banderas-Bravo E, et al. Replacement of 24-h creatinine clearance by 2-h creatinine clearance in intensive care unit patients: a single-center study. Intensive Care Med 2007;33(11):1900–6.
4. Kerl ME, Cook CR. Glomerular filtration rate and renal scintigraphy. Clin Tech Small Anim Pract 2005;20(1):31–8.
5. Prittie J, Langston C. Renal emergencies. In: Ettinger SJ, Feldman EC, editors. Textbook of veterinary internal medicine. 7th edition. St Louis (MO): Saunders Elsevier; 2010. p. 519–21.
6. Rodighiero V. Effects of liver disease on pharmacokinetics. An update. Clin Pharmacokinet 1999;37(5):399–431.
7. Zuppa AF, Barrett JS. Pharmacokinetics and pharmacodynamics in the critically ill child. Pediatr Clin North Am 2008;55(3):735–55, xii.
8. Shedlofsky SI, Israel BC, McClain CJ, et al. Endotoxin administration to humans inhibits hepatic cytochrome P450-mediated drug metabolism. J Clin Invest 1994; 94(6):2209–14.
9. Kirwan CJ, Lee T, Holt DW, et al. Using midazolam to monitor changes in hepatic drug metabolism in critically ill patients. Intensive Care Med 2009;35(7):1271–5.
10. Allegaert K, van Schaik RH, Vermeersch S, et al. Postmenstrual age and CYP2D6 polymorphisms determine tramadol o-demethylation in critically ill neonates and infants. Pediatr Res 2008;63(6):674–9.
11. Zagli G, Tarantini F, Bonizzoli M, et al. Altered pharmacology in the intensive care unit patient. Fundam Clin Pharmacol 2008;22(5):493–501.
12. Scaglione F, Paraboni L. Pharmacokinetics/pharmacodynamics of antibacterials in the intensive care unit: setting appropriate dosing regimens. Int J Antimicrob Agents 2008;32(4):294–301.
13. Parrillo JE. Pathogenic mechanisms of septic shock. N Engl J Med 1993;328: 1471–7.
14. Pea F, Porreca L, Baraldo M, et al. High vancomycin dosage regimens required by intensive care unit patients cotreated with drugs to improve haemodynamics following cardiac surgical procedures. J Antimicrob Chemother 2000;45(3): 329–35.
15. Parrillo JE, Parker MM, Natanson C, et al. Septic shock in humans. Advances in the understanding of pathogenesis, cardiovascular dysfunction, and therapy. Ann Intern Med 1990;113(3):227–42.
16. Marshall JC. Inflammation, coagulopathy, and the pathogenesis of multiple organ dysfunction syndrome. Crit Care Med 2001;29(Suppl 7):S99–106.
17. Posner LP, Burns P. Sedative agents: tranquilizers, alpha-2 agonists, and related agents. In: Riviere JE, Papich MG, editors. Veterinary pharmacology & therapeutics. 9th edition. Ames (IA): Wiley-Blackwell; 2009. p. 337–80.
18. Gehlbach BK, Kress JP. Sedation in the intensive care unit. Curr Opin Crit Care 2002;8(4):290–8.
19. Young CC, Prielipp RC. Benzodiazepines in the intensive care unit. Crit Care Clin 2001;17(4):843–62.
20. Kress JP, Pohlman AS, O'Connor MF, et al. Daily interruption of sedative infusions in critically ill patients undergoing mechanical ventilation. N Engl J Med 2000; 342(20):1471–7.
21. Young C, Knudsen N, Hilton A, et al. Sedation in the intensive care unit. Crit Care Med 2000;28(3):854–66.

22. Kukanich B, Papich MG. Opioid analgesic drugs. In: Riviere JE, Papich MG, editors. Veterinary pharmacology & therapeutics. 9th edition. Ames (IA): Wiley-Blackwell; 2009. p. 301–35.

23. Hall LG, Oyen LJ, Murray MJ. Analgesic agents. Pharmacology and application in critical care. Crit Care Clin 2001;17(4):899–923, viii.

24. Anand KJ, Barton BA, McIntosh N, et al. Analgesia and sedation in preterm neonates who require ventilatory support: results from the NOPAIN trial. Neonatal outcome and prolonged analgesia in neonates. Arch Pediatr Adolesc Med 1999; 153(4):331–8.

25. Adler MW, Geller EB, Rosow CE, et al. The opioid system and temperature regulation. Annu Rev Pharmacol Toxicol 1988;28:429–49.

26. Lucas AN, Firth AM, Anderson GA, et al. Comparison of the effects of morphine administered by constant-rate intravenous infusion or intermittent intramuscular injection in dogs. J Am Vet Med Assoc 2001;218(6):884–91.

27. Posner LP, Gleed RD, Erb HN, et al. Post-anesthetic hyperthermia in cats. Vet Anaesth Analg 2007;34(1):40–7.

28. Niedfeldt RL, Robertson SA. Postanesthetic hyperthermia in cats: a retrospective comparison between hydromorphone and buprenorphine. Vet Anaesth Analg 2006;33(6):381–9.

29. Golder FJ, Wilson J, Larenza MP, et al. Suspected acute meperidine toxicity in a dog. Vet Anaesth Analg 2010;37(5):471–7.

30. Hiraoka H, Yamamoto K, Okano N, et al. Changes in drug plasma concentrations of an extensively bound and highly extracted drug, propofol, in response to altered plasma binding. Clin Pharmacol Ther 2004;75(4):324–30.

31. Posner LP, Burns P. Injectable anesthetic agents. In: Riviere JE, Papich MG, editors. Veterinary pharmacology & therapeutics. 9th edition. Ames (IA): Wiley-Blackwell; 2009. p. 265–99.

32. Hay Kraus BL, Greenblatt DJ, Venkatakrishnan K, et al. Evidence for propofol hydroxylation by cytochrome P4502B11 in canine liver microsomes: breed and gender differences. Xenobiotica 2000;30(6):575–88.

33. Court MH, Hay-Kraus BL, Hill DW, et al. Propofol hydroxylation by dog liver microsomes: assay development and dog breed differences. Drug Metab Dispos 1999;27(11):1293–9.

34. Reid J, Nolan AM. Pharmacokinetics of propofol as an induction agent in geriatric dogs. Res Vet Sci 1996;61(2):169–71.

35. Ying SW, Goldstein PA. Propofol suppresses synaptic responsiveness of somatosensory relay neurons to excitatory input by potentiating GABA(A) receptor chloride channels. Mol Pain 2005;1:2.

36. Peeters MY, Aarts LP, Boom FA, et al. Pilot study on the influence of liver blood flow and cardiac output on the clearance of propofol in critically ill patients. Eur J Clin Pharmacol 2008;64(3):329–34.

37. Peeters MY, Bras LJ, DeJongh J, et al. Disease severity is a major determinant for the pharmacodynamics of propofol in critically ill patients. Clin Pharmacol Ther 2008;83(3):443–51.

38. Roberts JA, Lipman J. Pharmacokinetic issues for antibiotics in the critically ill patient. Crit Care Med 2009;37(3):840–51 [quiz: 859].

39. Marik PE. Aminoglycoside volume of distribution and illness severity in critically ill septic patients. Anaesth Intensive Care 1993;21(2):172–3.

40. Joynt GM, Lipman J, Gomersall CD, et al. The pharmacokinetics of once-daily dosing of ceftriaxone in critically ill patients. J Antimicrob Chemother 2001; 47(4):421–9.

41. Lipman J, Gous AG, Mathivha LR, et al. Ciprofloxacin pharmacokinetic profiles in paediatric sepsis: how much ciprofloxacin is enough? Intensive Care Med 2002; 28(4):493–500.

42. McKinnon PS, Paladino JA, Schentag JJ. Evaluation of area under the inhibitory curve (AUIC) and time above the minimum inhibitory concentration (T>MIC) as predictors of outcome for cefepime and ceftazidime in serious bacterial infections. Int J Antimicrob Agents 2008;31(4):345–51.

43. Georges B, Conil JM, Cougot P, et al. Cefepime in critically ill patients: continuous infusion vs. an intermittent dosing regimen. Int J Clin Pharmacol Ther 2005;43(8): 360–9.

44. Dahyot C, Marchand S, Bodin M, et al. Application of basic pharmacokinetic concepts to analysis of microdialysis data: illustration with imipenem muscle distribution. Clin Pharmacokinet 2008;47(3):181–9.

45. Joukhadar C, Frossard M, Mayer BX, et al. Impaired target site penetration of beta-lactams may account for therapeutic failure in patients with septic shock. Crit Care Med 2001;29(2):385–91.

46. Sauermann R, Delle-Karth G, Marsik C, et al. Pharmacokinetics and pharmacodynamics of cefpirome in subcutaneous adipose tissue of septic patients. Antimicrob Agents Chemother 2005;49(2):650–5.

47. Roberts JA, Roberts MS, Robertson TA, et al. Piperacillin penetration into tissue of critically ill patients with sepsis—bolus versus continuous administration? Crit Care Med 2009;37(3):926–33.

Goal-Directed Therapy in Small Animal Critical Illness

Amy L. Butler, DVM, MS

KEYWORDS

- Small animals • Critical illness • Early Goal-Directed Therapy
- Monitoring

Monitoring critically ill patients can be a daunting task even for experienced clinicians. Goal-directed therapy is a technique involving intensive monitoring and aggressive management of hemodynamics in patients with high risk of morbidity and mortality. The aim of goal-directed therapy is to ensure adequate tissue oxygenation and survival. This article reviews commonly used diagnostics in critical care medicine and what the information gathered signifies and discusses clinical decision making on the basis of diagnostic test results. One example is early goal-directed therapy for severe sepsis and septic shock. The components and application of goals in early goal-directed therapy are discussed.

MACROVASCULAR VERSUS MICROVASCULAR MONITORING PARAMETERS

To maintain homeostasis, adequate tissue and organ oxygenation must occur. Without adequate oxygen delivery and use, tissue hypoxia leads to cellular death, organ dysfunction, organ failure, and ultimately patient death. Potential causes of tissue hypoxia include failure of oxygen supply (macrocirculatory failure), failure of oxygen distribution (microcirculatory failure), and failure of oxygen processing (mitochondrial failure).[1]

The microcirculation is the network of vessels less than 100 microns in diameters, comprised of arterioles, capillaries, and venules. It is the largest endothelial surface in the body and is the site of oxygen, waste product, and nutrient exchange.[2] Flow through the microcirculation is controlled by local mediators, such as nitric oxide and the partial pressure of oxygen in the tissue (Po_2), as well as by the pressure gradient and resistance patterns created by the macrocirculation. Changes in systemic flow lead to changes in microcirculatory flow, which is subsequently adjusted for by local mediators.[3,4]

The question becomes, how does a clinician best monitor patients to ensure that all tissues are receiving adequate oxygenation? Monitoring parameters can best be

Veterinary Referral and Emergency Center, 318 Northern Boulevard, Clarks Summit, PA 18411, USA
E-mail address: abutler@vrecpa.com

Vet Clin Small Anim 41 (2011) 817–838
doi:10.1016/j.cvsm.2011.05.002
0195-5616/11/$ – see front matter © 2011 Elsevier Inc. All rights reserved.

divided into 2 broad categories: macrovascular and microvascular parameters.[5] Macrovascular parameters are related to systemic measures of cardiopulmonary status, such as blood pressure (BP), central venous pressure (CVP), and urine output. These are also referred to as upstream parameters, because they are measured before the tissue beds. Microvascular parameters are related to tissue oxygenation and include lactate and lactate clearance, central venous oxygen saturation ($S_{cv}O_2$), and base excess (BE).[6] These are also referred to as the downstream parameters, because they are measured after blood flows through the tissue beds. Addition experimental measures of microvascular flow include tissue specific tonometry, direct measurements of tissue P_{O_2}, tissue oximetry, laser Doppler, and sidestream dark-field microscopy.[7]

Of the tools listed, the macrovascular parameters are most commonly used by veterinarians. It is likely the health of the microcirculation, however, that determines tissue and organ survival, especially in critical illnesses, such as sepsis. Therefore, it is likely that monitoring a combination of both the macrocirculation and microcirculation provides the full spectrum of information required to make informed clinical decisions. Research into treatment bundles using both sets of parameters, especially those associated with early goal-directed therapy (EGDT) in sepsis, have shown that macrovascular and microvascular endpoints together are associated with significantly improved outcomes compared with any single endpoint alone.[8–11]

MACROVASCULAR MONITORING
Central Venous Pressure

The CVP is commonly used as an indicator of the volume status of a patient. The CVP is approximately equivalent to the right atrial pressure and thus right ventricular end diastolic pressure, which indicates the amount of preload available to the heart.[12] In theory, if the filling pressure of the heart is optimized, then cardiac output and thus oxygen delivery are maximized. CVP is easy to measure, but its use requires knowledge of inherent limitations.

The CVP is a measure of the hydrostatic pressure within the intrathoracic vena cava.[13] To be accurately measured, the catheter tip must be placed in the intrathoracic cranial vena cava[14] close to the right atrium. Both over-the-wire and through-the-needle catheters may be used for this purpose. Venous pressure measurements made from peripheral catheters have not been shown to correlate well with CVP measurements.[15] Once the catheter has been placed, the patient should placed in sternal or, ideally, lateral recumbency. It is important that patient position be the same for serial readings. A zero point should be chosen that corresponds with the level of the right atrium.[16] Either a water manometer or pressure transducer can be used for measurement of CVP, and values measured in millimeters of mercury can be converted to centimeters of water by multiplying by 1.36 (ie, 1 mm Hg = 1.36 cm H_2O). The normal reference range for dogs is 3.1 ± 4.1 cm H_2O.[17]

Although CVP is most often used as an estimate of volume status, many factors affect its measurement. False elevations in CVP can occur as a result of diastolic dysfunction, tricuspid regurgitation, decreased ventricular compliance, pulmonary hypertension, elevated intra-abdominal pressure, elevated intrathoracic pressure (as occurs with positive pressure ventilation), and pericardial effusion.[12] Some studies have suggested that CVP is a poor marker for intravascular volume.[18,19] Overall trends in CVP values are more likely to be of clinical use than a single measurement.[20,21] Generally speaking, a normal CVP does not necessarily indicate appropriate preload, and an abnormally low or high CVP should prompt additional investigation.[12]

If a previously normal CVP trends low, then the patient may be hypovolemic. A fluid challenge of isotonic crystalloid (10–20 mL/kg intravenously [IV]) or colloid (5 mL/kg IV) given over 5 to 10 minutes should cause an increase in CVP. If the CVP increases, then the patient is considered volume responsive. Patients who are responsive to crystalloid boluses may have a decrease in CVP as the fluid bolus redistributes to the interstitial space. In these cases, colloid infusions may be required to maintain an appropriate CVP, or higher crystalloid rates may be required. Many veterinarians aim for a CVP of 7 to 10 cm H_2O in critically ill patients. In human medicine, the EGDT guidelines for patients with septic shock recommend a target CVP of 8 to 12 mm Hg.[22] Conversely, a high CVP may indicate impending signs of volume overload. A high CVP should prompt a clinician to decrease fluid rates while also searching for one of the potential causes of falsely elevated CVP (listed previously). If no cause for false elevation can be found, then the clinician must assume that a high CVP is secondary to volume overload and reduce fluid rates and/or consider diuretic therapy. A low dose of furosemide (0.5 mg/kg IV or IM) should be considered in patients with evidence of pulmonary edema and should decrease the CVP over several hours provided that renal function is adequate.

A more challenging situation occurs when a high CVP is recorded in the face of low urine output. This typically indicates poor renal perfusion (from hypotension or renal artery thrombosis) or severe renal tubular or glomerular damage. Low intravascular volume is not likely the culprit, and patients with CVP greater than 10 mm Hg are less likely to respond to additional volume.[23] A high urine specific gravity (>1.035) may indicate poor renal perfusion, whereas a lower specific gravity may indicate acute renal failure. Another potential cause of elevated CVP with low urine output is syndrome of inappropriate secretion of antidiuretic hormone (SIADH), which has been reported in human patients as a result of neoplasia, central nervous system disease, intracranial disease, endocrine disease, postoperatively, and after administration of various drugs.[24] The hallmarks of SIADH include hyponatremia, impaired water excretion, hypo-osmolality, and high urine sodium concentrations.[25] Measurement of urine sodium concentrations may be beneficial. In human patients, a high urine sodium (>20 mEq/L) in combination with hyponatremia and hypoosmolality (<280 mOsm/L) suggest the presence of SIADH.[26] Reports in the veterinary literature are sparse, although SIADH has been reported as a result of central nervous sytem disease,[27,28] and elevated levels of ADH have been documented in the postoperative period.[29]

Blood Pressure

Arterial BP is the pressure exerted on the vascular walls and is derived from the ejection of blood from the left ventricle. The elastic distention of the arterial walls is responsible for maintenance of forward flow even during diastole. The mean arterial pressure (MAP) is not the average of the systolic and diastolic but instead represents the pressure in relation proportion of time spent in each phase of the cardiac cycle.

There are many different mechanisms of BP control, the discussion of which is beyond the scope of this article. Briefly, minute-to-minute BP control is under the governance of the sympathetic nervous system and circulating hormones, myogenic reflexes, and local feedback mechanisms. The primary site of BP control is the terminal and small arterioles.[30,31] Constriction of these arterioles leads to an increase in systemic BP at the expense of reduced flow to the capillary beds. This reduced flow is most pronounced in the hepatosplanchnic and skeletal muscle microcirculation, whereas autoregulation maintains flow in the cerebral, coronary, and renal circulations.

Because vasoconstriction or vasodilation may lead to changes in BP, a normal BP does not always imply normal tissue perfusion.

BP can be measured by invasive or noninvasive means. Direct arterial BP is measured by placement of a catheter into a peripheral artery. The dorsal pedal and femoral arteries are the most commonly used sites in clinical patients, although the radial, auricular, and coccygeal arteries can also be used. Once an arterial catheter is placed, it is connected via noncompliant, saline-filled tubing to a transducer, which translates the mechanical energy of the pressure waves into an electrical signal.[21] Direct arterial BP monitoring is considered the gold standard. Indications for direct BP monitoring include hemodynamic instability requiring beat-to-beat pressure measurement; the use of vasoactive substances, such as vasopressors or vasodilators; and requirement for frequent arterial blood sampling (pulmonary disease and ventilatory failure).

Major complications are rare, reported in less than 1% of human patients with arterial catheters.[32] The most common major complications include permanent ischemic damage, embolism, infection (local or systemic), or pseudoaneurysm. Minor complications, such as temporary occlusion, hematoma formation, or hemorrhage, can also occur. The major limiting factor for direct BP monitoring in veterinary medicine is the lack of appropriate equipment and the challenge of placing an arterial catheter in small patients.

The most common method of BP measurement in small animal medicine is through noninvasive BP (NIBP) monitoring. NIBP methods use a pressure cuff to occlude arterial blood flow, then either measure or allow detection of return of flow. Commonly used devices include the Dinamap, Cardell, Doppler, and high-definition oscillimetric systems. Standards for the validation of NIBP monitoring systems have been published for humans; however, none of these systems has met these criteria for dogs or cats.[33] Determining which device is most accurate for measurement of BP in dogs and cats has been a challenge in veterinary medicine.

Several recent studies have compared the accuracy of indirect BP measurements. One study compared Cardell, Passport, and Doppler NIBP with direct BP in conscious, critically ill dogs.[34] The investigators found that oscillimetric devices overestimated BP (compared with the direct method) in the hypotensive groups and were closer to the direct readings in the hypertensive group. Another study compared the petMap, an oscillimetric device, with direct pressures in hypotensive, anesthetized dogs.[35] Again, the NIBP overestimated BP in hypotensive patients. A similar study in anesthetized cats also showed poor agreement between veterinary-specific NIBP and direct pressures.[36] Overall, there is not one best NIBP monitor for use in critically ill veterinary patients because all tend to underestimate BP in hypotensive patients.

The recommendations for BP measurement in conscious dogs and cats come from the recent American College of Veterinary Internal Medicine consensus statement on monitoring of hypertension in dogs and cats.[33] The BP measurement should be performed in a quiet, isolated area after a patient has had time to adjust to its surroundings. The cuff should be 40% of the limb circumference in dogs and 30% to 40% of the limb circumference in cats. A too-small cuff artificially increases a reading, and a too-large cuff artificially decreases a reading. The first reading should be discarded, and the next 3 to 7 readings should be averaged. These readings should be consistent, with less than 20% variability in systolic values. Normal BP varies by species and breed. In dogs, normal systolic BP is approximately 140 mm Hg, with a normal diastolic pressure of 85 to 90 mm Hg. Normal mean BP in dogs is 100 mm Hg. Mean arterial pressure in greyhounds is approximately 20 mm Hg higher when compared with mongrel dogs.[37] In cats, systolic and diastolic BPs are normally 120 mm Hg and 80 mm Hg, respectively, with a MAP of 100 mm Hg.

Hypotension is defined as a MAP of less than 60 to 65 mm Hg. This is the range when renal and cerebral autoregulation are lost, and blood flow to these organs becomes dependent on systemic pressure. Hypotension is a common complication in critically ill patients and may be related to hypovolemia, other causes of inadequate cardiac output, or inappropriate vasodilation. Ideally, an arterial catheter and direct pressure monitoring should be performed in hypotensive critically ill patients or in any patients where hypotension may become a concern. Initially, volume responsiveness should be tested by giving a fluid challenge of 10 mL/kg to 22 mL/kg of isotonic crystalloids. If the BP responds to fluid resuscitation, additional volume may be required. Arterial BP measurements made in conjunction with CVP measurements can help a clinician decide if additional volume is needed. Fluid therapy should be titrated to effect; however, liberal fluid strategies are associated with development of edema and possibly a worse prognosis. In patients with sepsis, current recommendations are to volume load with crystalloid or colloids to a CVP of 8 to 12 cm H_2O.[38]

If patients are not responsive to fluid resuscitation, the next line of treatment for hypotension is the use of vasopressor agents. Inappropriate vasodilation is common in patients with sepsis or SIRS. This is due to lack of vascular responsiveness to catecholamines, depletion of vasopressin stores, or development of relative adrenal insufficiency. Commonly used vasopressors include dopamine, norepinephrine, vasopressin, and epinephrine. There is no evidence that one vasopressor is better than another for treatment of fluid-refractory hypotension in critical illness.[39,40] All pressors should be given as a constant rate infusion via a syringe pump.

- Dopamine is a precursor for norepinephrine and epinephrine and has dose-dependent effects. At low doses (0.5–2.0 µg/kg/min IV), it causes renal vasodilation without an increase in glomerular filtration rate and causes natriuresis by inhibiting Na+ transport in the renal tubules.[41] Its effects on urine output and so-called renal protection are controversial.[42–44] At medium doses (2–10 µg/kg/min IV), β_1-adrenergic effects are added to the dopaminergic effects, creating positive inotropy and increased cardiac output.[45] At higher doses (>10 mg/kg/min IV), mixed α-adrenergic and β-adrenergic effects predominate, creating a vasopressor effect.[46]
- Norepinephrine is a neurotransmitter and sympathetic catecholamine with mixed α and β adrenergic effects. Its primary site of activity is the α_1 receptor.[40] Doses range from 0.05 to 0.5 µg/kg/min IV, titrated to patient response. At least one study has found that norepinephrine was an effective rescue drug in human patients with hypotension refractory to other vasopressors.[47]
- Vasopressin is a hormone released from the posterior pituitary gland, with activity on numerous receptors. Activation of the V1 receptor, present on vascular smooth muscle, causes vasoconstriction.[48] Recommended doses in veterinary medicine vary. In one study, a dose of 0.5 to 1.25 mU/kg/min IV was recommended to treat dopamine-resistant vasodilatory shock.[49] The investigators in that study used doses of up to 5 mU/kg/min IV, with an average dose of 2.1 mU/kg/min IV. The current recommendation for dogs is a dose of 0.5 to 2.0 mU/kg/min IV.[50]
- Epinephrine is a potent α-adrenergic and β-adrenergic agonist, which causes vasoconstriction and increased cardiac output.[46] It can also cause increased tissue oxygen demand and severe splanchnic vasoconstriction, however, limiting its use to a second-line or third-line agent.[40] Long-term use is associated with tachyphylaxis. Doses range from 0.02 to 0.2 µg/kg/min IV.[45]

Realistically, the use of multiple vasopressors is associated with a poor prognosis for patients with critical illness. One study found that septic dogs with hypotension requiring pressor therapy after surgery were 2.35 times more likely to die than those without hypotension.[51] Another study of septic peritonitis in dogs found that patients receiving vasopressors (especially more than one vasopressor) were less likely to survive.[52] This does not imply a cause-and-effect relationship but does imply that dogs with severe enough disease to require vasopressor therapy were more likely to die.

Hypertension is less common in critically ill patients. Common nonpathologic causes for hypertension include pain, stress, and anxiety. Once those causes have been ruled out, systolic BPs greater than 180 mm Hg should be treated. Amlodipine (0.1–0.2 mg/kg by mouth up to every 4–6 hours as needed) or prazosin (1–4 mg total dose every 12 hours as needed) can be used. For severe, life-threatening hypertension, acepromazine, hydralazine, or sodium nitroprusside can be considered.

Urine Output

Acute kidney injury is a common complication in ICUs.[53] The term, acute kidney injury, encompasses the spectrum from minor changes in renal function to the need for renal replacement therapy.[54,55] In human medicine, the RIFLE criteria have been developed to define and classify renal injury.[55] The RIFLE classification system (Risk of renal dysfunction, Injury to the kidney, Failure of kidney function, Loss of kidney function and End-stage kidney disease) includes changes in serum creatinine, changes in glomerular filtration rate and/or changes in urine output. No such classification system currently exists in veterinary medicine.

Azotemia can be caused by renal, prerenal, or postrenal pathology. In general, renal azotemia is not evident until greater than 75% of renal function is lost, whereas loss of concentrating ability is not evident until greater than 66% of renal function is lost. In the face of normal hydration, oliguria is defined as urine output of less than 0.5 to 1.0 mL/kg/h, whereas anuria is defined as urine output of less than 0.3–0.5 mL/kg/h.[56] Conservative measures for prevention of AKI in critically ill patients include prevention of dehydration and hypotension and limiting exposure to nephrotoxicants, such as aminogylcosides, amphotericin and nonionic radiocontrast agents.[57]

Measuring urine output can easily be performed by placement of a urinary catheter. Alternatively, urine-soaked cage pads or blankets can be weighed to help determine production if a urinary catheter cannot be placed. Urine production less than 1 mL/kg/h should prompt the clinician to search for a possible cause. First, the urinary catheter should be checked for patency and positioning. The bladder can be assessed via manual palpation or ultrasound to determine if it is full. If the bladder is empty, the patient's hydration status should be assessed to rule out prerenal causes. It is important to recognize that hypovolemia may occur without evidence of external loss. Potential causes include gastrointestinal (GI) and respiratory losses, third spacing, increased vascular permeability, interstitial edema formation, and inappropriate vasodilation.[55] Hypotension or reduced cardiac output can also contribute to decreased urine output in the face of normovolemia.[53]

Although fluid therapy remains important, significant controversy exists over the most appropriate fluid choice, amount, and therapeutic goals when treating low urine output.[58] Overly aggressive fluid administration is currently thought detrimental.[59–62] In the face of clinically apparent overhydration, additional volume loading is not likely to improve urine production. Therefore, isotonic crystalloids should be cautiously administered in aliquots of 10 to 22 mL/kg if volume depletion is suspected. CVPs can help guide therapy, but at least one study has shown positive fluid balance in patients with normal CVPs, indicating that this monitoring tool is relatively insensitive.[63] Gains of 5% to 10% body weight are associated with positive fluid balance[62,64] and may be a better monitoring tool. All patients should be weighed at least once daily and ideally 2 to 3 times daily. Additionally, monitoring of urine for granular casts indicating tubular injury can be useful.[65]

If a patient appears clinically overhydrated or if a fluid challenge fails to improve urine output, the next step is to consider initiation of renal replacement therapies, such as intermittent hemodialysis or continuous renal replacement. Unfortunately, these treatment modalities are not widely available. Pharmacologic interventions may be attempted, such as renal-dose dopamine, furosemide, mannitol, fenoldopam, or diltiazem. Little evidence exists, however, to suggest that any of these improves renal recovery. Dopamine,[42,43] furosemide,[66,67] and mannitol[68] have been shown to create diuresis but have not been shown to improve survival or decrease the requirements for renal replacement therapies. In overhydrated patients, loop diuretics may reduce pulmonary edema and the need for mechanical ventilation. The use of fenoldopam and diltiazem is still under investigation. One study in healthy cats treated with fenoldopam showed an increase in urine output,[69] but no information is available on its use in critically ill animals. Diltiazem has been investigated in leptospirosis-induced renal failure in dogs and showed a trend toward but insignificant improvement in renal function.[70] Despite the lack of evidence, many clinicians use low doses of furosemide (0.1–0.5 mg/kg IV titrated or as a continuous rate infusion) as needed to induce diuresis in oliguric patients.

MICROVASCULAR MONITORING
Lactate and Lactate Clearance

Lactate is the product of pyruvate breakdown under anaerobic conditions. The majority of lactate production occurs in the GI tract and skeletal muscle, although brain, skin, and erythrocytes can contribute to production.[71] Circulating lactate is cleared by the liver. Two primary types of hyperlactatemia can occur, type A and type B (**Box 1**). Type A hyperlactatemia occurs when tissue oxygen delivery (Do_2) is insufficient to meet tissue demand (**Fig. 1**) and can be caused by shock, heart failure, local thromboembolism or torsion, hypoxemia, anemia, or exercise. Type B hyperlactatemia is not associated with tissue hypoxia but with insufficient lactate clearance (liver failure), abnormal mitochondrial function, certain drugs and toxins, or hypoglycemia.[72,73] Normal values for lactate in dogs have been reported to range from a mean of 1.11 mmol/L with the normal range up to 3.5 mmol/L,[74] with another study showing a mean lactate of 1.25 mmol/L, with a normal range of less than 2.5 mmol/L.[75] Normal values in cats are similar to dogs depending on the degree of struggling during sample collection.[76,77]

Lactate has been shown in many human[78–83] and veterinary studies to be an important prognostic indicator, likely because it reflects the degree of tissue dysoxia and the amount of physiologic stress. Previous veterinary literature has shown lactate of prognostic value in animals with SIRS,[84,85] babesiosis,[86] gastric dilatation-volvulus,[87] major trauma,[88] peritonitis,[89] and severe soft tissue infections.[90] Both human and veterinary researchers have concluded that the rate or effectiveness of lactate clearance is a more important prognostic marker[79,81,82,85] than a single initial measurement. This may be because the rate of lactate reduction reflects the rapidity of correction of tissue dysoxia.[73] Additionally, one study of dogs with SIRS showed no significant correlation between Do_2 and lactate.[84] Even at very low Do_2, lactate can be normal, although a high lactate level was usually associated with poor Do_2. The

Box 1
Causes of type A and type B hyperlactatemia

Type A Hyperlactatemia

- Tissue hypoperfusion
  - Hypovolemia (hemorrhage, severe dehydration)
  - Cardiogenic shock (myocardial failure, valvular disease, arrhythmias)
  - Obstructive shock (cardiac tamponade, arterial thromboembolism, GDV, mesenteric/colonic torsion)
  - Distributive shock (vasodilation, analophylaxis, sepsis)
- Severe anemia
- Severe hypoxemia
- Altered oxygen carrying states
  - Carboxyhemoglobin
  - Methemoglobin
- Excessive production
  - Tremors
  - Seizures
  - Exercise

Type B Hyperlactatemia

- Decreased clearance
  - Liver failure
- Abnormal oxygen utilization
  - Sepsis
  - SIRS
  - Diabetes mellitus
  - Renal failure
  - Neoplasia
  - Thiamine deficiency
  - Alkalemia
  - Short bowel syndrome
- Drugs/Toxins
  - Ethylene/Propylene glycol
  - Cathecholamines
  - Cyanide
  - Salicylates
  - Carbon monoxide
  - Nitroprusside
  - Acetaminophen
  - Terbutaline
  - Bicarbonate
  - Xylitol
  - Ethanol
- Congenital errors of metabolism

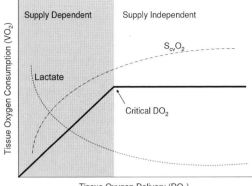

Fig. 1. Oxygen delivery versus consumption curve. Normal Do_2 is supply independent, meaning that oxygen delivery is in excess of tissue consumption. Once the critical DO_2 is reached, tissue oxygen consumption becomes dependent on delivery. In the supply-dependent portion of the curve, lactate levels increase as anaerobic metabolism increases and $S_{cv}o_2$ drops as the amount of oxygen extracted by the tissues increases.

conclusion was that although a high lactate is typically reflective of a low Do_2, a normal lactate does not mean that Do_2 is normal.

There are concerns with using lactate as a downstream marker for tissue perfusion in sepsis. Sepsis is associated with both type A and type B hyperlactatemia. Type A hyperlactatemia is most commonly caused by tissue hypoperfusion,[6,71] and septic states can create hypoperfusion through hypovolemia, cardiovascular derangements, and microvascular thrombosis.[91] Sepsis-related type B lactic acidosis can also occur through microvascular shunting and mitochondrial dysfunction.[92] Additionally, dysregulation of pyruvate dehydrogenase activity during sepsis can lead to increases in lactate concentrations.[93] Despite these concerns, lactate clearance has been shown to be a strong predictor of mortality in septic patients.[79,81]

In summary, two things are clear from previous lactate research: (1) the initial degree of hyperlactatemia does not seem to matter as much as the rate or effectiveness of clearance and (2) a normal lactate does not always indicate normal tissue perfusion.

Central Venous Oxygen Saturation

$S_{cv}o_2$ is a measure of the oxygenation of venous blood in the vena cava and is a reflection of tissue oxygen use. It can be used to monitor tissue perfusion and oxygen use.[6] $S_{cv}o_2$ is monitored via venous blood gases, co-oximetry, or continuous spectrophotometry. Pulse oximetry is not able to monitor $S_{cv}o_2$ because it requires pulsatile flow, and thus, can only be used for monitoring arterial oxygen saturations.

The $S_{cv}o_2$ reflects the balance of the amount Do_2 minus the amount extracted (Vo_2). In health, the amount of oxygen delivery to the tissues is far in excess of that which is needed (see **Fig. 1**). As the DO_2 decreases, through anemia, hypoxemia, or hypoperfusion, the percent of oxygen consumed, or the oxygen extraction ratio, increases to maintain tissue oxygenation.[94] In normal patients, $S_{cv}o_2$ is typically 65% to 75%.[95] In response to tissue dysoxia, the oxygen extraction ratio increases and the $S_{cv}o_2$ decreases. This results in maintenance of tissue oxygenation even in low flow states. The presence of a low $S_{cv}o_2$, however, also indicates ongoing tissue dysoxia and oxygen debt.[6]

The $S_{cv}o_2$ is often used as a surrogate for mixed venous oxygen saturation ($S_{mv}o_2$). The $S_{mv}o_2$ is drawn from a catheter placed within the pulmonary artery so that blood mixing from the cranial vena cava, caudal vena cava, and coronary circulation is included. The $S_{cv}O_2$ is usually drawn from a central line placed ideally within the cranial vena cava,[96] although the caudal vena cava can be used as well. Therefore, the $S_{cv}O_2$ reflects the organs draining the area from which the sample is being drawn (ie, a $S_{cv}O_2$ drawn from the cranial vena cava reflects the oxygen demand of the brain, head, and other cranial structures but does not reflect the oxygen demand of more caudal [abdominal] structures). The converse is true of samples drawn from the caudal vena cava. Neither $S_{cv}O_2$ drawn from the cranial nor caudal vena cava reflects coronary circulation. In healthy humans, $S_{cv}O_2$ is lower than $S_{mv}O_2$ by 2% to 3%, but in shock, the $S_{cv}O_2$ can exceed the $S_{mv}O_2$ by 8%.[97] There is considerable debate as to whether $S_{cv}O_2$ can be substituted for $S_{mv}O_2$.[98–100] $S_{mv}O_2$ and $S_{cv}O_2$ typically move in parallel,[101,102] however, and the most recent Surviving Sepsis Campaign guidelines judged them equivalent.[38]

$S_{cv}O_2$ has been shown to be a powerful predictor of tissue mortality in human patients,[103] especially in patients where normalization of $S_{cv}O_2$ cannot be attained.[104] No prospective studies have been published on association of $S_{cv}O_2$ with prognosis in veterinary medicine.

A low $S_{cv}O_2$ should prompt a clinician to first rule out hypotension and hypovolemia as potential causes for tissue hypoperfusion. An $S_{cv}O_2$ that remains low despite normalization of macrovascular parameters (heart rate, BP, and CVP) indicates ongoing tissue oxygen debt. Potential causes include decreased oxygen content (anemia or hypoxemia), decreased cardiac output, and inappropriate vasodilation. An arterial blood gas should be obtained, and supplemental oxygen administered if the patient is hypoxemic (Pao_2 <60 mm Hg). The hematocrit should be checked as well. In the guidelines for EGDT for sepsis,[22] the authors recommend transfusion of red blood cells to achieve a hematocrit of greater than 30% until $S_{cv}O_2$ is above 70%. This recommendation has been controversial due to known complications of blood transfusion, such as immunomodulation,[105,106] and the potential contribution to development of acute lung injury.[107,108] The need for blood transfusion should be balanced against the potential risks; however, continued low $S_{cv}O_2$ in a patient with a rapid drop in PCV is an indication for additional oxygen carrying capacity via blood transfusion.

If the $S_{cv}O_2$ does not respond to increased hematocrit, inotropic therapy with dobutamine is considered the next step. Dobutamine is a sympathomimetic with predominantly β_1-agonist effects, causing positive inotropy and chronotropy, increased stroke volume, and increased cardiac output.[109] The goal of dobutamine use is to increase forward flow in the hopes of improving perfusion. Doses range from 2 to 20 μg/kg/min IV as a constant rate infusion.

A high $S_{cv}O_2$ is less common but is also associated with abnormal tissue oxygenation. An $S_{cv}O_2$ greater than or equal to 80% is considered high and possibly represents impaired tissue oxygen extraction and use.[110] In septic patients, microcirculatory flow derangements and impaired mitochondrial function are known to reduce oxygen extraction.[5,92,111] There are no known interventions for high $S_{cv}O_2$, although a possible diagnosis of sepsis should be investigated in these patients.

Base Excess

BE is defined as the amount of base (or acid) in millimoles required to titrate the pH to 7.4 at normal body temperature (37°C), with a Pao_2 of 40 mm Hg. BE usually serves as a surrogate marker for metabolic acidosis because the Pao_2 is held constant. Metabolic acidosis has many causes, although lactic acidosis and accumulation of unmeasured acids can be caused by tissue hypoxia. Causes not related to ischemia are many and include renal failure, loss of bicarbonate through urine or diarrhea, and hyperchloremia.[112] It is important to differentiate between causes of ischemic and nonischemic acidosis. Although BE is thought to reflect lactate concentrations, this is not always true. Human studies have shown that BE may be poorly reflective of lactate.[113,114] A more strongly negative BE is associated with higher mortality in human studies.[115–117] In veterinary medicine, BE is associated with a worse prognosis in DKA[118] and is predictive of SIRS in dogs with pyometra.[119]

Despite its use as a prognostic tool, there is little information on how to use BE to guide therapy. A persistently low BE, especially in the face of normal lactate concentrations, should prompt a clinician to search for additional causes of metabolic acidosis.

ADVANCED MONITORING

New and experimental modalities are available for monitoring critically ill patients. These include cardiac output monitoring, tissue Po_2, sublingual capnography, sidestream dark-field microscopy, and tissue oximetry.

Early Goal-Directed Therapy

One of the best-defined examples for using monitoring to guide therapy is in human sepsis. EGDT for patients with severe sepsis and septic shock was first introduced by Rivers and colleagues[22] in 2001. The overall goal of EGDT is to match Do_2 with tissue oxygen demand to prevent pathologic supply dependence from developing. This is achieved by altering and optimizing the components of oxygen delivery (cardiac output and arterial oxygen content) and by reducing tissue oxygen demand (through sedation and mechanical ventilation). In their landmark article, Rivers and colleagues[22] demonstrated a 16% overall reduction in in-hospital mortality and a 12% reduction in 60-day mortality for the EGDT compared with the standard therapy group. On the basis of these findings, EGDT has been incorporated in the Surviving Sepsis Campaign as a "strong" recommendation,[38,120] is recommended by the Institute for Healthcare Improvement,[121] and is considered a quality indicator.[10,122]

EGDT is effective because it evaluates both macrovascular (upstream of tissue beds) and microvascular (downstream of tissue beds) parameters to allow the best evaluation of tissue perfusion possible.[6] The components of EGDT are as listed in **Fig. 2**.

The EGDT Bundle, Step-by-Step

Step 1: identification of a severe sepsis or septic shock patient

According to the American College of Chest Physicians and the Society of Critical Care Medicine (ACCP/SCCM), sepsis is defined as the systemic inflammatory response to an infection,[123] whether that is viral, bacterial, fungal, or protozoal infection. The systemic inflammatory response syndrome (SIRS) is a clinical syndrome composed of tachycardia, tachypnea, pyrexia, and alterations in white blood cell count. The presence of SIRS implies the presence of whole-body inflammation or systemic up-regulation of inflammatory mediators. SIRS criteria have been described for dogs[124] and cats,[125] although no consensus statement has been reached in the veterinary community.[126] Current criteria from Otto are listed in **Table 1**. When the presence of SIRS plus a documented (by culture, cytology, histopathology, or antigen testing) or strongly suspected infection exists, sepsis can be diagnosed.[123]

Severe sepsis and septic shock are subcategories of sepsis. Severe sepsis is defined as sepsis associated with organ dysfunction, perfusion abnormalities, or sepsis-induced hypotension.[123] Evidence of hypoperfusion includes increased blood

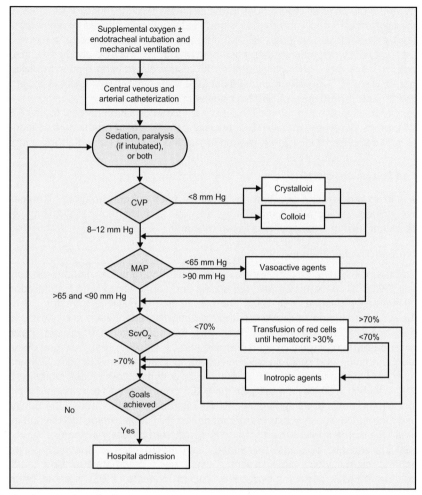

Fig. 2. The EGDT bundle. (*From* Rivers E, Nguyen B, Havstad S, et al. Early goal-directed therapy in the treatment of severe sepsis and septic shock. N Engl J Med 2001;345(19):1368–77; with permission.)

Table 1 SIRS criteria for dogs and cats[126]		
	Canine	**Feline**
Body temperature (°F)	<99.0; >103.0	<99.0; >103.0
Heart rate (beats/min)	>150	<140; >220
Respiratory rate (breath/min)	>40	>40
White blood cell count	<5000; >19,000 ± >5% bands	<5000; >20,000

Two or three of the four criteria must be present for diagnosis of SIRS.

lactate concentrations, evidence of organ dysfunction on biochemical analysis, or altered mentation. Septic shock is a subset of severe sepsis and is defined as sepsis-induced hypotension that is nonresponsive to adequate fluid therapy.[123] Septic shock is associated with signs of hypoperfusion (listed previously). Finally, multiple-organ dysfunction syndrome (MODS) can occur as the result of inflammation, coagulation, and altered endothelial function. MODS is defined by the ACCP/SCCM as alterations in organ function such that homeostasis cannot be maintained without intervention. Additional discussion of MODS is found elsewhere in this issue in the article by Timothy B. Hackett. Further definitions from the ACCP/SCCM consensus are listed in **Box 2**.

Step 2: identification of a high-risk patient

The high-risk patient is considered one that has a systolic BP less than 90 mm Hg after a 20-mL/kg to 40-mL/kg fluid challenge or has a lactate greater than 4 mmol/L. If a patient meets criteria for possible sepsis and is considered high risk, then instrumentation with a jugular central line and indwelling arterial catheter should be performed.

Step 3: target CVP of 8 to 12 mm Hg

The goal of this step is to increase intravascular volume. This can be accomplished by administration of isotonic crystalloids in aliquots of 10 to 22 mL/kg IV over 15 to 30 minutes up to a total volume of 80 to 90 mL/kg in dogs and 40 to 60 mL/kg in cats. Colloid preparations in aliquots of 5 mL/kg can be used as well, up to a total volume of 20 mL/kg. The choice of crystalloid, colloid, or both for volemic resuscitation in sepsis remains controversial.[127,128] The Surviving Sepsis Campaign guidelines do not recommend one fluid type over another.[38] It likely does not matter which fluid type is used, provided that adequate volumes are used.

Box 2

Definitions from the ACCP/SCCM consensus committee for sepsis and organ failure

- Infection: microbial phenomenon characterized by an inflammatory response to the presence of microorganisms or the invasion of normally sterile host tissue by those organisms

- Bacteremia: the presence of viable bacteria in the blood

- SIRS: the systemic inflammatory response to a variety of severe clinical insults as manifested by 2 or more of the following: tachycardia, tachypnea, pyrexia, and altered leukocyte count

- Sepsis: the systemic response to infection

- Severe sepsis: sepsis associated with organ dysfunction, hypoperfusion, or hypotension

- Septic shock: sepsis-induced hypotension despite adequate fluid resuscitation along with the presence of perfusion abnormalities

- Sepsis-induced hypotension: a systolic BP <90 mm Hg or a reduction of ≥40 mm Hg from baseline in the absence of other causes for hypotension

- MODS: presence of altered organ function in an acutely ill patient such that homeostasis cannot be maintained without intervention.

Data from Bone RC, Balk RA, Cerra FB, et al; ACCP/SCCM Consensus Conference Committee. Definitions for sepsis and organ failure and guidelines for the use of innovative therapies in sepsis. The ACCP/SCCM Consensus Conference Committee. American College of Chest Physicians/Society of Critical Care Medicine. 1992. Chest 2009;136(Suppl 5):e28.

Step 4: target MAP greater than 65 mm Hg and less than 90 mm Hg

BP should be monitored during fluid resuscitation. Often, hypotension reverses with administration of fluid alone. Monitoring of BP should ideally be performed with an indwelling arterial catheter and direct pressure measurement, especially if vasopressors or vasodilators are indicated after volume resuscitation. If fluid administration alone fails to increase BP, then vasopressor therapy should be initiated. In the original study, the vasopressor choice was left to the primary clinician. Currently, there is no overwhelming evidence to support the use of dopamine versus vasopressin versus norepinephrine over the others as a first-line vasopressor.[128–130] The Surviving Sepsis Campaign guidelines currently recommend either dopamine or norepinephrine as a first-line vasopressor.[38] Common vasopressor types and doses are listed elsewhere in this article.

Step 5: target $S_{cv}O_2$ greater than 70%

Once the goals in Steps 3 and 4 have been reached, a venous blood gas from the jugular central line should be obtained. If $S_{cv}O_2$ is not in the target range despite improvements in BP and CVP, then hematocrit should be assessed. If low, packed red blood cells should be transfused until the hematocrit is greater than 30%. This recommendation has been controversial[131] due to the aforementioned complications associated with blood transfusion. Currently, the Surviving Sepsis Campaign guidelines suggest, but do not recommend, transfusions.[38] For dogs, patients should be given type-specific blood and crossmatched if they have received prior transfusions. Feline patients should be given type-specific and crossmatched blood to avoid transfusion reactions.[132] As a rule of thumb, a dose of 1 mL/kg of packed red blood cells increases the PCV by 1%. If after transfusion, $S_{cv}O_2$ remains low, the use of dobutamine to increase cardiac output is recommended. The dose should be tirated upwards until the target $S_{cv}O_2$ is reached. If a patient becomes tachycardic or the MAP decreases to less than 65 mm Hg, the dobutamine dose should be decreased.[22]

Step 6: sedation and mechanical ventilation

If the goals of steps three through five cannot be reached despite patient optimization, then sedation and mechanical ventilation are indicated. The goal of this step is to decrease the patient oxygen demand.

Other Goals and Adjunctive Therapies for EGDT

Urine output greater than 0.5 mL/kg/h

During volume resuscitation, urine output should increase to greater than 0.5 mL/kg/h, especially as CVP goals are reached. If it does not, then the development of acute kidney injury should be considered. Fluid strategies and treatment are discussed previously.

Early source control

Every patient with possible sepsis should be evaluated for the presence of an infectious focus. Diagnostic work-up should proceed as a patient is stabilized. Biochemical profile and complete blood counts are indicated for all critically ill patients but do not always indicate the source of sepsis. Thoracic radiographs can be used to assess for the presence of radiographic patterns consistent with pneumonia or the presence of effusion associated with pyothorax. Abdominal ultrasound can be performed to look for the presence of free fluid indicating septic peritonitis or to look for potential intra-abdominal abscesses, pyometra, or prostatitis. Any peritoneal or pleural effusion present should be obtained via centesis and examined for the presence of white blood cells and intracellular bacteria. Paired lactate and glucose on the effusion and from the periphery can aid in diagnosis of septic effusions. Urinalysis and urine cultures should be obtained to rule out pyelonephritis. Cerebrospinal fluid and joint taps may be indicated if the source of infection cannot be found on initial diagnostic work-up. Bacterial translocation from the GI tract is a potential source of sepsis in patients with severe mucosal injury, especially those with parvovirus infections. The skin should be carefully checked for abscesses and infected wounds under the haircoat. If the source of sepsis is amenable to source control measures (such as surgical intervention), these should performed as soon as a patient is stabilized.

Early antibiotic therapy

Antibiotic therapy should be started as soon as sepsis is recognized. In humans with septic shock, mortality rates have been found to increase for every hour that antibiotic therapy is delayed.[133,134] Initiation of inappropriate antibiosis has also been associated with a 5-fold increase in mortality in human septic shock.[135] Cultures should ideally be obtained before starting, but should not delay, antibiotic therapy.[38] Broad-spectrum, combination antibiosis via the intravascular route is strongly recommended. Antibiotics should be bacteriocidal, not bacteriostatic. In veterinary medicine, combinations, such as enrofloxacin with ampicillin or ampicillin/sulbactam, or use with first-generation, second-generation, or third-generation cephalosporins are popular. The anaerobic spectrum can be extended with the addition of clindamycin or metronidazole if desired. Therapy with aminoglycosides should be avoided until a patient is fully hydrated and renal function has been assessed. Once culture results are available, antibiotic therapy should be de-escalated with the aim of using the most narrow-spectrum effective antibiotic.[128]

SUMMARY

Monitoring critically ill patients is a daunting task simply because of the large amount of diagnostic information required. The overall goal of goal-directed therapy is to ensure adequate tissue oxygenation to help improve tissue survival. The use of macrovascular and microvascular parameters together allows for the most complete assessment of patient status. Clinicians must be able to recognize, however, the indications and limitations of each test. Additionally, the presence of normal results does not necessarily mean normal tissue oxygenation. Instead, all information should be considered for the most accurate clinical assessment. Clinical decision making should be based on the known benefits and side effects of each treatment modality.

REFERENCES

1. Nencioni A, Trzeciak S, Shapiro N. The microcirculation as a diagnostic and therapeutic target in sepsis. Intern Emerg Med 2009;4(5):413–8.
2. Mohammed I, Norris S. Mechanisms, detection, and potential management of microcirculatory disturbances in sepsis. Crit Care Clin 2010;26(2):393–408.
3. Klijn E, Den Uil CA, Bakker J, et al. The heterogenity of the microcirculation in sepsis. Clin Chest Med 2008;29(4):643–54.
4. Elbers P, Ince C. Mechanisms of critical illness—classifying microcirculatory flow abnormalities in distributive shock. Crit Care 2006;10(4):221–9.
5. Trzeciak S, Rivers E. Clinical manifestations of disordered microcirculatory perfusion in severe sepsis. Crit Care 2005;9(S4):S20–6.
6. Prittie J. Optimal endpoints of resuscitation and early goal-directed therapy. J Vet Emerg Crit Care 2006;16(4):329–39.

7. DeBacker D, Ospina-Tascon G, Salgado D, et al. Monitoring the microcirculation in the critically ill patient: current methods and future approaches. Intensive Care Med 2010;36:1813–25.

8. Barochia A, Cui X, Vitberg D, et al. Bundled care for septic shock: an analysis of clinical trials. Crit Care Med 2010;38(2):668–78.

9. Levy MM, Dellinger RP, Townsend SR, et al. The Surviving Sepsis Campaign: results of an international guideline-based performance improvement program targeting severe sepsis. Intensive Care Med 2010;36(2):222–31.

10. Nguyen HB, Corbett SW, Steele R, et al. Implementation of a bundle of quality indicators for the early management of severe sepsis and septic shock is associated with decreased mortality. Crit Care Med 2007;35(4):1105–12.

11. Ramos FJ, Azevedo L. Hemodynamic and perfusion end points for volemic resuscitation in sepsis. Shock 2010;34(S1):34–9.

12. Gelman S. Venous function and central venous pressure. Anesthesiology 2008; 108(4):735–48.

13. Aldrich J, Haskins S. Monitoring the critically ill patient. In: Bonagura J, Kirk R, editors. Current veterinary therapy. Philadelphia: WB Saunders; 1995. p. 98–105.

14. Hayashi Y, Maruyama K, Takaki O, et al. Optimal placement of CVP catheter in paediatric cardiac patients. Can J Anaesth 1995;46(6):479–82.

15. Chow R, Kass P, Haskins S. Evaluation of peripheral and central venous pressure in awake dogs and cats. Am J Vet Res 2006;67(12):1987–91.

16. Laforcade AD, Rozanski E. Central venous pressure and arterial blood pressure measurements. Vet Clin North Am Small Anim Pract 2001;31(6):1163–74.

17. Haskins S, Pascow PJ, Ilkiw JE, et al. Reference cardiopulmonary values in normal dogs. Comp Med 2005;55(2):156–61.

18. Lichtwarck-Aschoff M, Beale R, Pfeiffer U. Central venous pressure, pulmonary artery occlusion pressure, intrathoracic blood volume, and right ventricular end-diastolic volume as indicators of cardiac preload. J Crit Care 1996; 11(4):180–8.

19. Wiesenack C, Fiegl C, Keyser A, et al. Continuously assessed right ventricular end-diastolic volume as a marker of cardiac preload and fluid responsiveness in mechanically ventilated cardiac surgical patients. Crit Care 2005;9(3): R226–33.

20. Dalrymple P. Central venous pressure monitoring. Anaesth Intensive Care 2006; 7(3):91–2.

21. Barbeito A, Mark J. Arterial and central venous pressure monitoring. Anesthesiol Clin 2006;24(4):717–35.

22. Rivers E, Nguyen B, Havstad S, et al. Early goal-directed therapy in the treatment of severe sepsis and septic shock. N Engl J Med 2001;345(19): 1368–77.

23. Magder S, Bafaqeeh F. The clinical role of central venous pressure measurement. J Intensive Care Med 2007;22(1):44–51.

24. Hannon M, Thompson C. The syndrome of inappropriate antidiuretic hormone: prevalence, causes and consequences. Eur J Endocrinol 2010;162(S1):S5–12.

25. Kovacs L, Robertson G. Syndrome of inappropriate antidiuresis. Endocrinol Metab Clin North Am 1992;21(4):859–75.

26. Patel G, Balk R. Recognition and treatment of hyponatremia in acutely ill hospitalized patients. Clin Ther 2007;29(2):211–29.

27. Shiel R, Pinilla P, Mooney C. Syndrome of inappropriate antidiuretic hormone secretion associated with congenital hydrocephalus in a dog. J Am Anim Hosp Assoc 2009;45(5):249–52.

28. Brofman P, Knostman K, DiBartola S. Ganulomatous amebic meningoencephalitis causing the syndrome of inappropriate secretion of antidiuretic hormone in a dog. J Vet Intern Med 2003;17(2):230–4.
29. Hauptman J, Richter MA, Wood SL, et al. Effects of anesthesia, surgery and intravenous administration of fluids on antidiuretic hormone concentrations in healthy dogs. Am J Vet Res 2000;61(10):1273–6.
30. Segal S. Regulation of blood flow in the microcirculation. Microcirculation 2005; 12(1):33–45.
31. Bevan J. Control of peripheral vascular resistance: evidence based on the in vitro study of resistance arteries. Clin Invest Med 1987;10(6):568–72.
32. Scheer B, Perel A, Pfeiffer U. Clinical review: complications and risk factors of peripheral arterial catheters used for haemodynamic monitoring in anaesthesia and intensive care medicine. Crit Care 2002;6(3):198–204.
33. Brown S, Atkin C, Bagley R, et al. Guidelines for the identification, evaluation and management of systemic hypertension in dogs and cats. J Vet Intern Med 2007;21(3):542–58.
34. Bosiack AP, Mann FA, Dodam JR, et al. Comparison of ultrasonic Doppler flow-monitor, oscillometric, and direct arterial blood pressure measurements in ill dogs. J Vet Emerg Crit Care 2010;20(2):207–15.
35. Shih A, Robertson S, Vigani A, et al. Evaluation of an indirect oscillimetric blood pressure monitor in normotensive and hypotensive anesthetized dogs. J Vet Emerg Crit Care 2010;20(3):313–8.
36. Acierno M, Seaton D, Mitchell MA, et al. Agreement between directly measured blood pressure and pressures obtained with three veterinary-specific oscillometric units in cats. J Am Vet Med Assoc 2010;237:402–6.
37. Cox R, Peterson L, Detweiler D. Comparison of arterial hemodynamics in the mongrel dog and the racing greyhound. Am J Physiol 1976;230(1):211–8.
38. Dellinger RP, Levy MM, Carlet JM, et al. Surviving Sepsis Campaign: international guidelines for management of severe sepsis and septic shock: 2008. Crit Care Med 2008;36(1):296–327.
39. Mullner M, Urbanek B, Havel C, et al. Vasopressors for shock. Cochrane Database Syst Rev 2004;3:CD003709.
40. Shapiro D, Loiacono L. Mean arterial pressure: therapeutic goals and pharmacologic support. Crit Care Clin 2010;26(2):285–93.
41. Schenarts P, Sagraves SG, Bard MR, et al. Low-dose dopamine: a physiologically based review. Curr Surg 2006;63(3):219–25.
42. Lauschke A, Teichgraber UK, Frei U, et al. 'Low-dose' dopamine worsens renal perfusion in patients with acute renal failure. Kidney Int 2006;69:1669–74.
43. Bellomo R, Chapman M, Finfer S, et al. Low-dose dopamine in patients with early renal dysfunction: a placebo-controlled randomised trial. Lancet 2000; 356:2139–43.
44. Kellum J, Decker J. Use of dopamine in acute renal failure: a meta-analysis. Crit Care Med 2001;29(8):1526–31.
45. Long K, Kirby R. An update on cardiovascular adrenergic receptor physiology and potential pharmacological applications in veterinary critical care. J Vet Emerg Crit Care 2008;18(1):2–25.
46. Wohl J, Clark T. Pressor therapy in critically ill patients. J Vet Emerg Crit Care 2000;10(1):21–34.
47. Jhanji S, Stirling S, Patel N, et al. The effect of increasing doses of norepinephrine on tissue oxygenation and microvascular flow in patients with septic shock. Crit Care Med 2009;37:1961–6.

48. Scroggin R, Quandt J. The use of vasopressin for treating vasodilatory shock and cardiopulmonary arrest. J Vet Emerg Crit Care 2009;19(2):145–57.

49. Silverstein D, Waddell LS, Drobatz KJ, et al. Vasopressin therapy in dogs with dopamine-resistant hypotension and vasodilatory shock. J Vet Emerg Crit Care 2007;17(4):399–408.

50. Silverstein D. Vasopressin. In: Silverstein D, Hopper K, editors. Small animal critical care medicine. St Louis (MO): Saunders Elsevier; 2009. p. 759–62.

51. Kenney E, Rozanski EA, Rush JE, et al. Association between outcome and organ system dysfunction in dogs with sepsis: 114 cases (2003–2007). J Am Vet Med Assoc 2010;236(1):83–7.

52. Bentley A, Otto C, Shofer F. Comparison of dogs with septic peritonitis: 1988–1993 versus 1999–2003. J Vet Emerg Crit Care 2007;17(4):391–8.

53. Kellum J. Acute kidney injury. Crit Care Med 2008;36(4S):S141–5.

54. Mehta R, Kellum JA, Shah SV, et al. Acute Kidney Injury Network: report of an initiative to improve outcomes in acute kidney injury. Crit Care 2007;11(3):R31.

55. Bellomo R, Ronco C, Kellum JA, et al. Acute renal failure—definition, outcome measures, animal models, fluid therapy and information technology needs: the Second International Consensus Conference of the Acute Dialysis Quality Initiative (ADQI) Group. Crit Care 2004;8(2):R204–12.

56. Srisawat N, Hoste E, Kellum J. Modern classification of acute kidney injury. Blood Purif 2010;29(3):520–4.

57. Venkataraman R. Can we prevent acute kidney injury? Crit Care Med 2008; 36(4S):S166–71.

58. Bagshaw S, Bellomo R, Kellum JA. Oliguria, volume overload and loop diuretics. Crit Care Med 2008;36(4S):S172–8.

59. Cerda J, Sheinfeld G, Ronco C. Fluid overload in critically ill patients with acute kidney injury. Blood Purif 2010;29(4):331–8.

60. Bagshaw S, Brophy PD, Cruz D, et al. Fluid balance as a biomarker: impact of fluid overload on outcome in critically ill patients with acute kidney injury. Crit Care 2008;12(4):169.

61. Bouchard J, Soroko SB, Chertow GM, et al. Fluid accumulation, survival and recovery of kidney function in critically ill patients with acute kidney injury. Kidney Int 2009;76(4):422–7.

62. Payen D, de Pont AC, Sakr Y, et al. A positive fluid balance is associated with a worse outcome in patients with acute renal failure. Crit Care 2008;12(3): R74–81.

63. Schrier R. Fluid administration in critically ill patients with acute kidney injury. Clin J Am Soc Nephrol 2010;5(4):733–9.

64. Prowle J, Echeverri JE, Ligabo EV, et al. Fluid balance and acute kidney injury. Nat Rev Nephrol 2010;6:107–15.

65. Kanbay M, Kasapoglu B, Perazella M. Acute tubular necrosis and pre-renal acute kidney injury: utility of urine microscopy in their evaluation- a systematic review. Int Urol Nephrol 2010;42(2):425–33.

66. Ho K, Sheridan D. Meta-analysis of frusemide to prevent or treat acute renal failure. Br Med J 2006;333(7565):420.

67. Bagshaw S, Delaney A, Haase M, et al. Loop diurectics in the the management of acute renal failure: a systematic review and meta-analysis. Crit Care Resusc 2007;9(1):60–8.

68. Solomon R, Werner C, Mann D, et al. Effects of saline, mannitol, and furosemide to prevent acute decreases in renal function induced by radiocontrast agents. N Engl J Med 1994;331(21):1416–20.

69. Simmons J, Wohl JS, Schwartz DD, et al. Diuretic effects of fenoldopam in healthy cats. J Vet Emerg Crit Care 2006;16(2):96–103.

70. Mathews K, Monteith G. Evaluation of adding diltiazem therapy to standard treatment of acute renal failure cause by leptospirosis: 18 dogs (1998–2001). J Vet Emerg Crit Care 2007;17(2):149–58.

71. Lagutchik MS, Ogilvie GK, Wingfield WE, et al. Lactate kinetics in veterinary critical care: a review. J Vet Emerg Crit Care 1996;6(2):81–95.

72. Karagiannis MH, Reniker AN, Kerl ME, et al. Lactate measurement as an indicator of perfusion. Comp Cont Educ Pract Vet 2006;28(4):287–99.

73. Pang DS, Boysen S. Lactate in veterinary critical care: pathophysiology and management. J Am Anim Hosp Assoc 2007;43(5):270–9.

74. Evans G. Plasma lactate measurements in healthy beagle dogs. Am J Vet Res 1987;48(1):141–2.

75. Hughes D, Rozanski ER, Shofer FS, et al. Effect of sampling site, repeated sampling, pH, and PCO2 on plasma lactate concentration in healthy dogs. Am J Vet Res 1999;60(4):521–4.

76. Christopher MM, O'Neill S. Effect of specimen collection and storage on blood glucose and lactate concentrations in healthy, hyperthyroid and diabetic cats. Vet Clin Pathol 2000;29(1):22–8.

77. Rand JS, Kinnaird E, Baglioni A, et al. Acute stress hyperglycemia in cats is associated with struggling and increased concentrations of lactate and norepinephrine. J Vet Intern Med 2002;16(2):123–32.

78. Husain FA, Martin MJ, Mullenix PS, et al. Serum lactate and base deficit as predictors of mortality and morbidity. Am J Surg 2003;185(5):485–91.

79. Arnold RC, Sahpiro NI, Jones AE, et al. Multicenter study of early lactate clearance as a determinant of survival in patients with presumed sepsis. Shock 2009; 32(1):35–9.

80. Jones AE, Shapiro NI, Trzeciak S, et al. Lactate clearance vs central venous oxygen saturation as goals of early sepsis therapy: a randomized clinical trial. JAMA 2010;303(8):739–46.

81. Nguyen HB, Rivers EP, Knoblich BP, et al. Early lactate clearance is associated with improved outcome in severe sepsis and septic shock. Crit Care Med 2004; 32(8):1637–42.

82. Donnino MW, Miller J, Goyal N, et al. Effective lactate clearance is associated with improved outcome in post-cardiac arrest patients. Resuscitation 2007; 75(2):229–34.

83. Kamolz L, Andel H, Schramm W, et al. Lactate: early predictor of morbidity and mortality in patients with severe burns. Burns 2005;31(8):986–90.

84. Butler A, Campbell VL, Wagner AE, et al. Lithium dilution cardiac output and oxygen delivery in conscious dogs with systemic inflammatory response syndrome. J Vet Emerg Crit Care 2008;18(3):248–57.

85. Stevenson CK, Kidney BA, Duke T, et al. Serial blood lactate concentrations in systemically ill dogs. Vet Clin Pathol 2007;36(3):234–9.

86. Nel M, Lobetti RG, Keller N, et al. Prognostic value of blood lactate, blood glucose, and hematocrit in canine babesiosis. J Vet Intern Med 2004;18(4):471–6.

87. de Papp E, Drobatz KJ, Hughes D. Plasma lactate concentration as a predictor of gastric necrosis and survival among dogs with gastric dilatation-volvulus: 102 cases (1995–1998). J Am Vet Med Assoc 1999;215(1):49–52.

88. Gower SB, Weisse CW, Brown DC. Major abdominal evisceration injuries in dogs and cats: 12 cases (1998–2008). J Am Vet Med Assoc 2009;234(12): 1566–72.

89. Parsons KJ, Owen LJ, Lee K, et al. A retrospective study of surgically treated cases of septic peritonitis in the cat (2000–2007). J Small Anim Pract 2009; 50(10):518–24.

90. Buriko Y, Van Winkle TJ, Drobatz KJ, et al. Severe soft tissue infections in dogs: 47 cases (1996–2006). J Vet Emerg Crit Care 2008;18(6):608–18.

91. Jones AE, Puskarich MA. Sepsis-induced tissue hypoperfusion. Crit Care Clin 2009;25(4):769–79.

92. Fink M. Bench-to-bedside review: cytopathic hypoxia. Crit Care 2002;6(6):491–9.

93. Thomas GW, Mains CW, Slone DS, et al. Potential dysregulation of the pyruvate dehydrogenase complex by bacterial toxins and insulin. J Trauma 2009;67(3): 628–33.

94. Muir W. Trauma: physiology, pathophysiology, and clinical implications. J Vet Emerg Crit Care 2006;16(4):253–63.

95. Rady M, Rivers E, Nowak RM. Resuscitation of the critically ill in the ED: responses of blood pressure, heart rate, shock index, central venous oxygen saturation, and lactate. Am J Emerg Med 1996;14(2):218–25.

96. Kissoon N, Spenceley N, Krahn G, et al. Continuous central venous oxygen saturation monitoring under varying physiological conditions in an animal model. Anaesth Intensive Care 2010;38(5):883–9.

97. Marx G, Reinhart K. Venous oximetry. Curr Opin Crit Care 2006;12(3):263–8.

98. Chawla L, Zia H, Gutierrez G, et al. Lack of equivalence between central and mixed venous oxygen saturation. Chest 2004;126(6):1891–6.

99. Lorentzen A, Lindshov C, Sloth E, et al. Central venous oxygen saturation cannot replace mixed venous saturation in patients undergoing cardiac surgery. J Cardiothorac Vasc Anesth 2008;22(6):853–7.

100. Martin C, Auffray JP, Badetti C, et al. Monitoring of central venous oxygen saturation versus mixed venous oxygen saturation in critically ill patients. Intensive Care Med 1992;18(2):101–4.

101. Dueck M, Klimek M, Appenrodt S, et al. Trends but not individual values of central venous oxygen saturation agree with mixed venous oxygen saturation during varying hemodynamic conditions. Anesthesiology 2005;103(2):249–57.

102. Pérez A, Eulmesekian PG, Minces PG, et al. Adequate agreement between venous oxygen saturation in right atrium and pulmonary artery in critically ill children. Pediatr Crit Care Med 2009;10(1):76–9.

103. Pope J, Jones AE, Gaieski DF, et al. Multicenter study of central venous oxygen saturation (ScvO2) as a predictor of mortality in patients with sepsis. Ann Emerg Med 2010;55(1):40–6.

104. Lima A, van Bommel J, Jansen TC, et al. Low tissue oxygen saturation at the end of early goal-directed therapy is associated with worse outcome in critically ill patients. Crit Care 2009;13(S5):S13.

105. Vamvakas E, Blajchman M. Transfusion-related immunomodulation (TRIM): an update. Blood Rev 2007;21(6):327–48.

106. Vamvakas E, Blajchman M. Transfusion-related mortality: the ongoing risks of allogeneic blood transfusion and the available strategies for their prevention. Blood 2009;113(15):3406–17.

107. Marik P, Corwin H. Acute lung injury following blood transfusion: expanding the definition. Crit Care Med 2008;36(11):3080–4.

108. Swanson K, Dwyre DM, Krochmal J, et al. Transfusion-related acute lung injury (TRALI): current clinical and pathophysiologic considerations. Lung 2006; 184(3):177–85.

109. Beale R, Hollenberg SM, Vincent JL, et al. Vasopressor and inotropic support in septic shock: an evidence based review. Crit Care Med 2004;2004(32):S11.

110. Perz S, Uhlig T, Kohl M, et al. Low and "supranormal" central venous oxygen saturation and markers of tissue hypoxia in cardiac surgery patients: a prospective observational study. Intensive Care Med 2011;37(1):52–9.

111. DeBacker D, Creteur J, Preiser JC, et al. Microvascular blood flow is altered in patients with sepsis. Am J Respir Crit Care Med 2002;166(1):98–104.

112. Englehart M, Schreiber M. Measurement of acid-base resuscitation endpoints: lactate, base deficit, bicarbonate or what? Curr Opin Crit Care 2006;12(6): 259–574.

113. Chawla L, Jagasia D, Abell LM, et al. Anion gap, anion gap corrected for albumin, and base deficit fail to accurately diagnose clinically significant hyperlactatemia in critically ill patients. J Intensive Care Med 2008;23(2):122–7.

114. Park M, Azevedo LC, Maciel AT, et al. Evolutive standard base excess and serum lactate level in severe sepsis and septic shock patients resuscitated with early goal-directed therapy: still outcome markers? Clinics (Sao Paulo) 2006;61(1):47–52.

115. Surbatovic M, Radakovic S, Jevtic M, et al. Predictive value of serum bicarbonate, arterial base deficit/excess and SAPS III score in critically ill patients. Gen Physiol Biophys 2009;28(Spec No):271–6.

116. Rixen D, Raum M, Bouillon B, et al. Base deficit development and its prognostic significance in posttrauma critical illness: an analysis by the trauma registry of the Deutsche Gesellschaft für unfallchirurgie. Shock 2001;15(2):83–9.

117. Rutherford E, Morris JA, Reed GW, et al. Base deficits stratifies mortality and determines therapy. J Trauma 1992;33(3):417–23.

118. Hume D, Drobatz K, Hess R. Outcome of dogs with diabetic ketoacidosis: 127 dogs (1993–2003). J Vet Intern Med 2006;20(3):547–55.

119. Hagman R, Reezigt BJ, Bergstrom Ledin H, et al. Blood lactate levels in 31 female dogs with pyometra. Acta Vet Scand 2009;51:2–12.

120. Dellinger RP, Carlett JM, Masur H, et al. Surviving Sepsis Campaign guidelines for management of severe sepsis and septic shock. Crit Care Med 2004;32(3): 858–73.

121. Levy MM. Severe sepsis bundles. Institute for Healthcare Improvement. Available at: www.IHI.org/IHI/Topics/CriticalCare/Sepsis. Accessed December 13, 2010.

122. Schorr C. Performance improvement in the management of sepsis. Crit Care Clin 2009;25(4):857–67, x.

123. Bone RC, Balk RA, Cerra FB, et al; ACCP/SCCM Consensus Conference Committee. Definitions for sepsis and organ failure and guidelines for the use of innovative therapies in sepsis. The ACCP/SCCM Consensus Conference Committee. American College of Chest Physicians/Society of Critical Care Medicine. 1992. Chest 2009;136(Suppl 5):e28.

124. Hauptman JG, Walshaw R, Olivier NB. Evaluation of the sensitivity and specificity of diagnostic criteria for sepsis in dogs. Vet Surg 1997;26(5):393–7.

125. Brady CA, Otto CM. Systemic inflammatory response syndrome, sepsis, and multiple organ dysfunction. Vet Clin North Am Small Anim Pract 2001;31(6): 1147–62, v–vi.

126. Otto CM. Sepsis in veterinary patients: what do we know and where can we go? J Vet Emerg Crit Care 2007;17(4):329–32.

127. Bozza F, Carnevale R, Japiassu AM, et al. Early fluid resuscitation in sepsis: evidence and perspectives. Shock 2010;34(S1):40–3.

128. Raghavan M, Marik P. Management of sepsis during the early "golden hours". J Emerg Med 2009;31(2):185–99.
129. Holmes C, Walley K. Vasoactive drugs for vasodilatory shock in ICU. Curr Opin Crit Care 2009;15(5):398–402.
130. Povoa P, Carneiro A. Adrenergic support in septic shock: a critical review. Hosp Pract 2010;38(1):62–73.
131. Otero R, Nguyen HB, Huang DT, et al. Early goal-directed therapy in severe sepsis and septic shock revisited. Chest 2006;130(5):1579–95.
132. Weinstein N, Blais MC, Harris K, et al. A newly recognized blood group in domestic shorthair cats: the Mik red cell antigen. J Vet Intern Med 2007;21(2): 287–92.
133. Gaieski DF, Mikkelsen ME, Band RA, et al. Impact of time to antibiotics on survival in patients with severe sepsis or septic shock in whom early goal-directed therapy was initiated in the emergency department. Crit Care Med 2010;38(4):1045–53.
134. Kumar A, Roberts D, Wood KE, et al. Duration of hypotension before initiation of effective antimicrobial therapy is the critical determinant of survival in human septic shock. Crit Care Med 2006;34(6):1589–95.
135. Kumar A, Ellis P, Arabi Y, et al. Initiation of inappropriate antimicrobial therapy results in a fivefold reduction of survival in human septic shock. Chest 2009; 136(5):1237–48.

Index

Note: Page numbers of article titles are in **boldface** type.

A

N-Acetylcysteine, in hepatic dysfunction management, 755
Activated partial thromboplastin time, coagulation defects and, 787–788
Activated protein C, for coagulation defects, 792–793
Acute kidney injury (AKI), RIFLE classification scheme for, 733
Acute liver failure (ALF). See also *Hepatic dysfunction.*
    CNS dysfunction in, 749–750
    described, 745
    in dogs and cats, causes of, 746, 747
    risk factors for, 750–751
Acute lung injury (ALI)
    critical illness and, 712
    treatment of, 712–714
Acute Physiology and Chronic Health Evaluation II scoring system, 705
Acute renal failure (ARF)
    AKI and, 733–734
    causes of, 734–736
    community-acquired, 735
    defined, 733
    early detection of, 738–739
    hospital-acquired, 735–736
        prevention of, 737–739
            risk factor awareness in, 737
            risk factor management in, 737–738
    management of, 739–742
    normotensive ischemic, 737
    pathophysiology of, 734
Acute respiratory distress syndrome (ARDS)
    critical illness and, 709
    pathophysiology of, 712
    treatment of, 712–714
S-Adenosylmethionine (SAMe), in hepatic dysfunction management, 753–755
AKI. See *Acute kidney injury (AKI).*
ALF. See *Acute liver failure (ALF).*
ALI. See *Acute lung injury (ALI).*
Analgesia/analgesics, for gastrointestinal dysfunction due to critical illness in
    small animals, 764
Antibacterials, in critical care setting, 812
Antibiotics, for gastrointestinal dysfunction due to critical illness in small animals, 763
Antiemetics, for gastrointestinal dysfunction due to critical illness in small animals, 764
Antioxidants, in hepatic dysfunction management, 753–755
Antithrombin, coagulation defects and, 789, 791–792

Vet Clin Small Anim 41 (2011) 839–846
doi:10.1016/S0195-5616(11)00115-X
0195-5616/11/$ – see front matter © 2011 Elsevier Inc. All rights reserved.
vetsmall.theclinics.com

ARDS. See *Acute respiratory distress syndrome (ARDS).*
ARF. See *Acute renal failure (ARF).*
Arginine, for gastrointestinal dysfunction due to critical illness in small animals, 763–764
Ascites, in hepatic dysfunction, 748–749
Autonomic impairment, in sepsis and critical illness, 722–723
Azotemia
    approach to, clinical questions related to, 731
    defined, 728
    prerenal, renal, and postrenal, differentiation among, 729–731
    renal failure and, 728–731

B

Bacterial translocation, 760
Base excess, in microvascular monitoring in goal-directed therapy in critically ill animals,
    826–827
Benzodiazepines, in critical care setting, 810–811
Blood pressure, in macrovascular monitoring in goal-directed therapy in critically ill
    animals, 819–822

C

Cardiovascular system
    critical illness effects on, **717–726**
        drug disposition and therapeutic response related to, 810
    sepsis effects on, **717–726**. See also *Sepsis, cardiovascular dysfunction in.*
Cat(s), ALF in, causes of, 746, 747
Central nervous system (CNS), dysfunction of, in ARF, 749–750
Central venous oxygen saturation, in microvascular monitoring in goal-directed therapy in
    critically ill animals, 825–826
Central venous pressure, in macrovascular monitoring in goal-directed therapy in critically
    ill animals, 818–819
Chronic kidney disease (CKD)
    defined, 732
    staging of, 732
CIRCI. See *Critical illness–related corticosteroid insufficiency (CIRCI).*
CKD. See *Chronic kidney disease (CKD).*
CNS. See *Central nervous system (CNS).*
Coagulation
    defects in
        activated partial thromboplastin time and, 787–788
        antithrombin and, 789
        detection of, platelet function assays in, 788–789
        diagnosis of, 786–787
        fibrinolysis assessment in, 789
        in critical illness, **783–803**
        microparticles and, 788
        platelet count and, 787
        protein C activity and, 789
        prothrombin and, 787–788
        treatment of, 790–795

activated protein C in, 792–793
antithrombin in, 791–792
fresh frozen plasma in, 790–791
heparin in, 793–795
platelet transfusion in, 793
vitamin K in, 795
viscoelastic coagulation monitoring of, 788
inflammation effects on, 783–784
intravascular thrombosis and, 784–785
Community-acquired acute renal failure, 735
Critical illness. See also specific types.
cardiovascular dysfunction in, 717–726. See also Sepsis, cardiovascular dysfunction in.
corticosteroid insufficiency due to, 767–782. See also Critical illness–related corticosteroid insufficiency (CIRCI).
drug metabolism alterations during, 805–815
drugs used in, 810–812. See also specific drugs.
gastrointestinal dysfunction due to, 759–766. See also Gastrointestinal dysfunction.
goal-directed therapy in, 817–833. See also Goal-directed therapy, in critically ill animals.
kidney in, 727–744. See also Kidney(s), critical illness effects on.
physiologic alterations in
drug disposition effects of, 808–810
therapeutic response effects of, 808–810
respiratory complications of, 709–716. See also Respiratory disorders, complications associated with, critical illness and.
Critical illness–related corticosteroid insufficiency (CIRCI), 767–782
clinical signs of, 774–775
diagnosis of, 775–777
incidence of, 770–774
syndrome of, described, 767–768
treatment of, 777–778

D

Diarrhea, hemorrhagic, critical illness in small animals and, 760–761
DIC. See Disseminated intravascular coagulation (DIC).
Disseminated intravascular coagulation (DIC). See also Coagulation, defects in.
coagulation defects and, 783–784
described, 783–784
treatment of, 789–790
Dog(s)
ALF in, causes of, 746, 747
cardiac performance in septic shock in, 718–719
Drug disposition, physiologic alterations in critical illness effects on, 808–810
Drug metabolism, alterations of, in critically ill animals, 805–815. See also specific drugs.

E

Early goal-directed therapy (EGDT)
adjunctive therapies for, 830–831
goals of, 830–831
in critically ill animals, 827–831

Early goal-directed therapy (EGDT) bundle, in critically ill animals, step-by-step approach, 827–830

EGDT. See *Early goal-directed therapy (EGDT)*.

Electrolyte abnormalities, in hepatic dysfunction, 748–749

Endothelial cell damage, MODS and, 712

F

Fibrinolysis, assessment of, coagulation defects and, 789

Fluid therapy, for gastrointestinal dysfunction due to critical illness in small animals, 762

Flumazenil, in hepatic dysfunction management, 754

Fresh frozen plasma, for coagulation defects, 790–791

G

Gastrointestinal dysfunction
bacterial translocation and, 760
critical illness in small animals and, **759–766,** 809–810
diagnostic evaluation of, 761–762
drug disposition and therapeutic response related to, 809–810
hemorrhagic diarrhea, 760–761
prognosis of, 764
symptoms of, 759
treatment of
analgesics in, 764
antibiotics in, 763
antiemetics in, 764
arginine in, 763–764
fluid therapy in, 762
glutamine in, 763
omega-3 fatty acid supplementation in, 763–764
symptomatic, 762
Gastrointestinal tract, defense mechanisms of, 760
Glucocorticoid(s), reduced access to target tissues and cells during illness, 770
Glucocorticoid synthesis, decreased, during illness, 768–770
Glutamine, for gastrointestinal dysfunction due to critical illness in small animals, 763
Glutathione, in hepatic dysfunction management, 754–755
Goal-directed therapy, in critically ill animals, **817–833**
advanced monitoring in, 827–831
early, 827–831
macrovascular monitoring in
blood pressure, 819–822
central venous pressure, 818–819
urine output, 822–823
vs. microvascular monitoring, 817–818
microvascular monitoring in
base excess, 826–827
central venous oxygen saturation, 825–826
lactate and lactate clearance, 823–825

H

Heart rate, in sepsis and critical illness, 722–723
Hemorrhagic diarrhea, critical illness in small animals and, 760–761
Hemostasis
 metabolic disease and, 786
 trauma and, 785–786
Heparin, for coagulation defects, 793–795
Hepatic dysfunction, **745–758**
 defined, 745–746
 diagnosis of, 751–753
 indicators of, 751–753
 manifestations of
  ascites, 748–749
  electrolyte abnormalities, 748–749
 prognosis of, 756
 risk factors for, 750–751
 sepsis and, 746–748
 treatment of, 753–755
  N-acetylcysteine in, 755
  antioxidants in, 753–755
  goals of, 753
  milk thistle in, 755
  SAMe in, 753–755
  vitamin E in, 755
Hospital-acquired acute renal failure, 735–736
 prevention of, 737–739
Hypothalamic-pituitary-adrenal (HPA) axis
 abnormal response of, during illness, 768–770
 activation of, 767
 normal regulation of, during illness, 768

I

Immunity, innate, toll-like receptors and, in sepsis and critical illness, 720
Inflammation, coagulation effects of, 783–784
Innate immunity, toll-like receptors and, in sepsis and critical illness, 720
Intravascular thrombosis, coagulation effects of, 784–785

K

Kidney(s)
 critical illness effects on, **727–744**
  drug disposition and therapeutic response related to, 808–809
 normal functions of, 727–728
Kidney disease. See also *Acute renal failure (ARF)*.
 in critically ill small animals, **727–744**
  chronic disease, definition and staging of, 732

L

Lactate, in microvascular monitoring in goal-directed therapy in critically ill animals, 823–825

Lactate clearance, in microvascular monitoring in goal-directed therapy in critically ill animals, 823–825

Lactulose, in hepatic dysfunction management, 754

Liver
    critical illness effects on, drug disposition and therapeutic response related to, 809
    dysfunction of, **745–758.** See also *Hepatic dysfunction.*

M

Mannitol, in hepatic dysfunction management, 754

Metabolic disease, hemostatic defects secondary to, 786

Metronidazole, in hepatic dysfunction management, 754

Microparticles, coagulation defects and, 788

Milk thistle, in hepatic dysfunction management, 755

MODS. See *Multiple organ dysfunction syndrome (MODS).*

MOF. See *Multiple organ failure (MOF).*

Multiple Organ Dysfunction Score, 705

Multiple organ dysfunction syndrome (MODS)
    adverse effects of, 712
    clinical scoring systems for, 705
    defined, 703
    diagnostic evaluation of, 705–706
    endothelial cell damage due to, 712
    epidemiology of, 704
    history of, 703–704
    introduction to, **703–707**
    pathophysiology of, 704–705

Multiple organ failure (MOF). See also *Multiple organ dysfunction syndrome (MODS).*
    defined, 703
    history of, 703–704
    introduction to, **703–707**

Myocardial depression, in sepsis and critical illness, 722–723

Myocardial dysfunction
    cascade of events from trigger to, 721–722
    sepsis-induced, mechanisms of, 719

N

Neomycin, in hepatic dysfunction management, 754

Normotensive ischemic acute renal failure, 737

O

Omega-3 fatty acid supplementation, for gastrointestinal dysfunction due to critical illness in small animals, 763–764

Opioid(s), in critical care setting, 811

P

Pharmacokinetics, described, 805–808

Platelet count, coagulation defects and, 787

Platelet function assays, in coagulation defects detection, 788–789
Platelet transfusion, for coagulation defects, 793
Propofol, in critical care setting, 811–812
Protein C, activated, for coagulation defects, 792–793
Protein C activity, coagulation defects and, 789
Prothrombin, coagulation defects and, 787–788

R

Relative adrenal insufficiency. See *Critical illness–related corticosteroid insufficiency (CIRCI)*.
Renal failure
    acute. See *Acute renal failure (ARF)*.
    azotemia and, 728–731
    uremia and, 728–731
Renal function
    normal, 727–728
    worsening, signs of, 728
Respiratory disorders, complications associated with, critical illness and, **709–716**
    ALI, 712
    ARDS, 709
    prevalence of, 709
    SIRS, 709–712

S

SAMe. See *S-Adenosylmethionine (SAMe)*.
Sepsis
    ACCP/SCCM consensus conference definitions of, 710
    autonomic impairment associated with, 722–723
    cardiovascular dysfunction in, **717–726**
        cascade of events from trigger to myocardial dysfunction, 721–722
        heart rate–related, 722–723
        myocardial depression, 722–723
        myocardial dysfunction, mechanisms of, 719
        septic shock, 717–719
        therapeutic potentials, 723–724
        toll-like receptors and innate immunity, 720
    critical illness and, 709–712
    hepatic manifestations of, 746–748
    stages of, 711
Septic shock, cardiac performance in, 717–719
    in dogs, 718–719
    in humans, 717–718
Sequential Organ Failure Assessment, 705
Shock, septic. See *Septic shock*.
SIRS. See *Systemic inflammatory response syndrome (SIRS)*.
Sonoclot, 788
Systemic inflammatory response syndrome (SIRS), to infection, 710

T

TEG. See *Thromboelastography (TEG)*.
Therapeutic response, physiologic alterations in critical illness effects on, 808–810

Thrombocytopenia, causes of, 787
Thromboelastography (TEG), 788
Thrombosis(es), intravascular, coagulation effects of, 784–785
Toll-like receptors, innate immunity and, in sepsis and critical illness, 720
Transfusion, platelet, for coagulation defects, 793
Translocation, bacterial, 760
Trauma, hemostasis and, 785–786

U

Uremia
    defined, 728
    renal failure and, 728–731
Urine output, in macrovascular monitoring in goal-directed therapy in critically ill animals,
    822–823

V

Viscoelastic coagulation monitoring, 788
Vitamin E, for hepatic dysfunction, 755
Vitamin K, for coagulation defects, 795

Moving?

Make sure your subscription moves with you!

To notify us of your new address, find your **Clinics Account Number** (located on your mailing label above your name), and contact customer service at:

Email: journalscustomerservice-usa@elsevier.com

800-654-2452 (subscribers in the U.S. & Canada)
314-447-8871 (subscribers outside of the U.S. & Canada)

Fax number: 314-447-8029

Elsevier Health Sciences Division
Subscription Customer Service
3251 Riverport Lane
Maryland Heights, MO 63043

*To ensure uninterrupted delivery of your subscription, please notify us at least 4 weeks in advance of move.